THE
HOSPITAL
SAFETY
DIRECTOR'S
HANDBOOK

Second Edition

Kenneth S. Weinberg BA, MSc, PhD

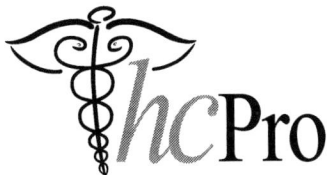

*hc*Pro

The Hospital Safety Director's Handbook, Second Edition, is published by HCPro, Inc.

Copyright 2003 by HCPro, Inc.

HCPro, Inc., provides information resources for the health care industry.

HCPro, Inc., is not affiliated in any way with the Joint Commission on Accreditation of Healthcare Organizations (JCAHO), which owns the JCAHO trademark.

Kenneth S. Weinberg, BA, MSc, PhD, Author
Judith Kelliher, Managing Editor
Kelly Ahlquist, Copy editor
Mike Mirabello, Senior Graphic Artist
Matthew Sharpe, Graphic Artist
Tom Philbrook, Cover Designer
Bob Croce, Group Publisher
Jean St. Pierre, Creative Director
Suzanne Perney, Publisher

Advice given is general. Readers should consult professional counsel for specific legal, ethical, or clinical questions. Arrangements can be made for quantity discounts.

For more information on this or any other HCPro, Inc., publication, contact:

HCPro, Inc.
P.O. Box 1168
Marblehead, MA 01945
Telephone: 800/650-6787 or 781/639-1872
Fax: 781/639-2982
E-mail: customerservice@hcpro.com

Visit HCPro, Inc., at its World Wide Web sites:
www.hcmarketplace.com, www.hcpro.com, and www.accreditinfo.com

11/2003
18352

Contents

About the Author

Kenneth S. Weinberg, BA, MSc, PhD

Kenneth S. Weinberg, BA, MSc, PhD, is president and principal consultant of Safdoc Systems, LLC, based in Stoughton, MA. Safdoc specializes in environmental health and safety and toxicology.

Weinberg's extensive experience in health care and health care safety includes serving as director of safety at Massachusetts General Hospital (MGH) in Boston for more than 10 years. He also held the post of assistant safety officer at MGH for 18 months prior to serving as director. He also worked as an industrial hygienist in a Veteran's Administration hospital in the Boston area.

Weinberg is a professional member of the American Society of Safety Engineers (ASSE) and for two years was the administrator of its HealthCare Division. In addition, he is listed in the National Registry of Safety Professionals and is a registered professional industrial hygienist. He is a Certified Toxics Use Reduction Planner for general practice. In 2001, the Healthcare Specialty Practice of ASSE at its annual Professional Development Conference named Weinberg Safety Professional of the Year.

Weinberg's educational background and training includes a bachelor's degree in biology from Boston University, a master's degree in environmental health and radiation health physics from the University of Pittsburgh Graduate School of Public Health, and a doctorate in biochemistry and pathology from Boston University Graduate School's Division of Medical and Dental Sciences.

Prior to reentry into safety and industrial hygiene, Weinberg's work dealt with pulmonary disease and the study of the causes of various pulmonary diseases, including cancer by environmental pollutants.

In addition to his consulting work, Weinberg teaches, writes articles for professional journals, and speaks during conferences and seminars around the country. He is an editor of several national safety publications, and has contributed chapters for books on health and safety.

Weinberg has authored two books, the first edition of *The Hospital Safety Director's Handbook*, and *Indoor Air Quality During Construction: A Guide to Best Engineering Practices and Regulatory Compliance*, both published by HCPro.

Acknowledgments

The opportunity to put to paper your experiences and to share them with your colleagues is very special. The chance to update those ideas and share them a second time is even more special and a wonderful privilege.

At the same time, the writing, preparation, and editing of the text requires a great deal of help and patience from a number of people. I want to thank Bob Croce of HCPro, Inc., for yet another chance to write a book specifically designed for safety directors in health care. I also want to thank the editor of this book, Judy Kelliher, for her ideas, comments, and insightful questions. I also want to thank Bob and Judy for their patience with me.

The last person I wish to thank is the first person in my heart, and the one who is always there to help and support me, Natalie, my wife.

Chapter 1

The Safety Director

The role of the safety director

As safety director, you fill a dynamic role in the hospital. You continuously monitor for potential hazards and maintain a system-wide safety program, sending a message to patients, staff, and the community that the hospital is safe and environmentally sound. In monitoring for hazards, you must determine its potential exposures. Following are some general environmental health and safety (EH&S) action points for you:

- Take precautions against undesirable chemical, biological, and radiation exposures to staff, patients, and visitors. Update regularly policies and procedures affecting these areas. Continuously train staff. Verify that equipment is in safe working order. Consider modern treatments and therapies that take place everyday in the typical hospital: No doubt there are potentially thousands of safety issues.

- Watch for contaminated needles. Train staff in the latest safety measures to prevent needlesticks and to safely dispose of used needles. At the same time, reassure patients that the hospital is expert at taking precautions with needles and other medical supplies.

- Consider the community's fear for the environment because of effluents from your hospital's air stacks or the solid, infectious, chemical, or radioactive waste it may produce.

- Maintain fire safety as it historically has been one of the first areas of concern for hospitals because many patients may be nonambulatory or restrained by their medical conditions or treatment.

- Educate staff about proper lifting techniques as injuries to employees from repeated stress trauma has taken the spotlight over the past several years. Back and neck injuries are a major source of reportable injuries and account for significant lost work time among nursing staff. Develop polices and procedures to help reduce and prevent the occurrence of such injuries.

- Maintain involvement with nurses, administrators, construction personnel, and infection control practitioners by performing preconstruction risk assessments. Risk assessments conducted in the planning stages of a construction or renovation project are now required by the Joint Commission on Accreditation of Healthcare Organizations (JCAHO) as well as the American Institute of Architects and the Centers for Disease Control and Prevention (CDC). They are designed to identify potential sources of harm to patients so that steps can be taken to prevent any adverse events from occurring.

- Get the facts about indoor air quality and develop policies and procedures to deal with employee complaints. More than at any time in the past, public buildings—hospitals among them—have been more proactive in their response to patient and employee complaints about indoor air quality problems. Many of the issues surrounding indoor air quality are rooted in the energy crisis of the 1970s when buildings were built to ensure that costs for energy could be kept low. By the 1990s, hospital workers, like the general public, were very aware of the indoor air quality problems that they might encounter in their place of work. In response to the onslaught of complaints, safety directors found that they needed to become more educated about the causes of these problems and their solutions. Hospitals also needed to develop policies and procedures to deal with employee complaints about indoor air.

• Collaborate with purchasing agents, glove manufacturers, and others who have had to develop and implement programs that introduce substitute products for gloves containing a high amount of latex. The emergence of HIV and AIDS in the early 1980s resulted in massive increases in the use of latex gloves because they provided the best protection of workers against possible infection by this deadly virus. By the late '80s and early '90s, many health care workers found that they were allergic to latex. As many as 8% to 10% of health care workers are now recognized as being allergic to latex. This latex allergy presented some major concerns and problems both for health care workers and the hospitals that employ them.

• Step up preparations and plans for dealing with wide-scale accidents and/or terrorist attacks involving the use of biological weapons. Hospitals have always been required to be prepared to participate in community drills in preparation for any disastrous event that would adversely affect the community, the hospital, and its ability to provide medical care to its patients or to the large numbers of injured persons who would come to them seeking medical care. In light of the events of September 11, 2001, there has been a renewed concern and awareness on the part of hospitals of the need to be prepared for community-wide disasters or terrorist attacks.

As the previous list shows, a hospital's safety needs vary dramatically. You must cast a wide net to monitor all potential exposure. Gone are the days when you would maintain only a fire prevention program. While many of the accreditation standards from the Joint Commission revolve around having a strong fire safety program—and fires remain a serious concern for patient and employee safety—fire safety should be just one component of a comprehensive EH&S program. Many potential hazards have existed for years; it is only recently that the health care industry has become aware of these hazards.

Does every hospital need a safety director?

The hospital administrator must decide whether someone should be designated as safety director. In the early 1980s, the Joint Commission took note of the significant rise of injuries among health care workers. In response to this increase, the JCAHO strongly suggested, but did not mandate, that all health care facilities should have a person or group of persons responsible for safety at their facilities.

The decision to appoint someone as the safety director should take into account the JCAHO's recommendation but, more important, should be based on the hospital's potential exposures regarding EH&S and the regulatory requirements the hospital must meet. Remember, safety and environmental hazards exist in every hospital, and every hospital must be prepared to deal with them.

Although some hospitals succeed in divvying up the various EH&S duties among several employees, it is paramount that one person—be it the safety director or someone else in the organization—is responsible for the overall program.

To some degree, the position of hospital safety director exists not only because of internal risks but also because of public and regulatory perceptions. Public and private agencies have campaigned to spread awareness of the potential risks of working in or living near a hospital. No longer is a hospital readily accepted as a benevolent and welcome member of the community. Instead, a hospital is viewed like any other company that must be regulated, controlled, and monitored.

Local, state, and federal agencies are interested in hospitals and how they provide for employee safety and community well-being. The Occupational Safety and Health Administration (OSHA) and the Environmental Protection Agency (EPA) realize that hospitals are one of the major employers in America and that they are full of potential hazards. Since the mid 1980s, regulations on hazard communication, use of personal protective equipment, reduction of toxic air emissions, and disposal of hazardous waste have been applied as rigorously and uniformly to the health care industry as to any other industry.

Because of the potential for HIV transmission and tuberculosis (TB) exposure to health care workers, OSHA directs many regulations exclusively to hospitals and other health care facilities. In addition, the mounting levels of mercury in fish have resulted in regulations aimed at curbing hospital use and disposal of mercury by local water authorities and the EPA. Hospitals, in turn, have responded to these regulations. Many have instituted programs to eliminate mercury and products containing mercury, such as thermometers or sphygmomanometers. You provide the leadership for these programs.

In recognition of safety risks, the JCAHO has updated its requirements and expectations about hospital worker safety and environmental health. Standards today encompass Environment of Care (EC), which is an effort to review, evaluate, and monitor all aspects of occupational and EH&S.

A hospital chooses to assign a safety director for a number of reasons. Above all, it needs a safety director on staff who is a:

- professional with knowledge in EH&S matters
- professional who allows the hospital to focus all safety issues in one area of responsibility
- leader who can develop and manage programs designed to reduce employee injuries
- knowledgeable person who can work with staff to help them better understand and comply with a myriad of regulatory requirements
- professional who is up-to-date on all EH&S issues that have an impact on the hospital
- professional who can use his or her skills to effectively educate employees about the potential hazards they face on the job

Who are safety directors?

A hospital's safety director should have experience in EH&S oversight and should be trained in the workings of a hospital. In addition, this person would benefit from a background in the scientific and regulatory requirements needed to ensure worker safety and environmental health. Experience could also include workplace evaluations, protective equipment, techniques for monitoring chemical exposures, and knowledge in environmental regulations. (See Figure 1.1 for a sample job description.)

Figure 1.1

Sample Safety Director Job Description

Usually the job description for the individual responsible for EH&S is a very broad, open-ended document. This is in recognition that the field is evolving quickly. Health care is discovering many new areas of responsibility open to safety directors. Therefore, room must be left for expansion of the safety director's duties so that the document doesn't have to be rewritten. For example, some of the new areas of responsibility include elimination of mercury from the hospital environment, compliance with Clean Air Act emissions requirements, and toxic waste reduction. The job description for the person charged with EH&S might look something like this:

The safety director

- reports directly to the president about all matters relating to EH&S issues. In compliance with all local, state, and federal requirements, he or she works in conjunction with the safety committee to develop and maintain an environment that is safe for employees, patients, and visitors.

Figure 1.1

Sample Safety Director Job Description (cont.)

- reviews, develops, and updates safety policies and procedures as needed, but no less often than annually. The manager ensures that all employees are educated and trained on how to perform their tasks in a safe manner. He or she provides necessary information to ensure that all workers are knowledgeable about hospital safety procedures, including, but not limited to, safety procedures for dealing with all hazardous materials, wastes, chemicals, sharps, and cytotoxic drugs.

- conducts surveillance rounds in all areas of the hospital at least twice a year. He or she is also responsible for reporting all issues, problems, and concerns to the safety committee on a routine basis. He or she will report all emergent issues to the president, as deemed necessary. In conjunction with the safety committee, the safety director will assist department heads and supervisors in eliminating or resolving safety issues.

- interacts with all regulatory agencies and files all reports on safety and environmental issues.

- monitors any and all potential employee exposures to hazardous chemicals, such as formaldehyde or ethylene oxide, or any other chemical requiring such monitoring.

- monitors chemical or waste releases to the environment, including, but not limited to, air or water effluents.

- oversees all hazardous chemical waste disposals. He or she is also responsible for maintaining the records for these activities.

All other items not mentioned specifically but that may evolve relating to EH&S will be assigned, as required, to the safety director.

The educational background of safety directors varies, but typically they have a focus in the sciences or engineering. The fields of study could include biology, chemistry, physics, or engineering. The American Society of Safety Engineers and the American Industrial Hygiene Association—two of the most prominent professional organizations for EH&S—have upgraded their requirements for credentialing to include both bachelor's and master's degrees.

What to expect as safety director

As the safety director, you will face many challenges from all parts of the hospital. Everyone from the person who loads the laundry into the truck for shipment off to the cleaner up to the president of the hospital or the hospital legal counsel will be calling to ask for your advice or input on one matter or another. Sometimes the questions and the challenges will be simple. At other times the questions will be challenging, requiring you to use all your resources, experience, and training to come up with a solution to a difficult problem. For example:

- How do you propose to get the ventilation system back in working order without having to order an evacuation of one of the most critical patient care areas in the hospital?
- Did the leak above the ceiling expose anyone to harmful chemicals or biological agents?
- Can the pregnant woman continue to work in the laboratory where they are storing the radium implants?

There are, of course, the routine, day-to-day tasks such as conducting surveillance rounds, monitoring employee exposures to chemicals, or presenting a

Chapter 2

Getting Organized

Congratulations! Your organization has just put you in charge of EH&S. You'll be the first safety director in your organization's history. Until now, individuals carried out EH&S matters as they saw fit, typically reacting to EH&S concerns as they developed within various departments. You know that major changes are needed, but what's the most effective way to bring them about?

One of the first things to do is advise the president or chief executive officer (CEO) that the organization needs a safety committee. The safety committee will lend you support and structure as you manage EH&S.

Putting together your safety committee

Some consider a safety committee a necessary evil; although working with a safety committee can seem burdensome and time-consuming, it can also help you achieve your goals more thoroughly and quickly than you could if left to your own devices. Moreover, your job is so all-encompassing that you need a committed and active safety committee to do it effectively.

Several elements will decide whether your committee will be successful. Perhaps foremost is the selection of committee members. The committee chair typically has the last word in the choice, but his or her selection is subject to the approval of the president or CEO. As the safety director, take part in the selection process. Consider the following 10 individuals for the safety committee:

1. **Department heads** or supervisors are responsible already for safety issues in their areas.

2. **Staff members** and employees are often interested in EH&S issues.

3. **Hospital administration** should be represented on the committee. This sends a message that the highest levels of the organization endorse the committee and will give it necessary financial support.

4. **Engineering, housekeeping, and hospital police or security** department members will be good allies and can help you quickly resolve many safety-related problems.

5. **Nurses** are typically the largest segment of your health care staff. You'll need their support.

6. **Clinical and research laboratory representatives** can give essential input as many safety issues arise in these areas.

7. **Physicians** often are overlooked when it comes to EH&S. They are greatly involved in hospital affairs and should be represented on the safety committee.

8. Representatives from **radiation safety, occupational health, and infection control** interact with safety regularly and safety committee issues frequently will cross over these disciplines.

9. **Unions** are typically required for any safety-related negotiations, and having them on the committee can facilitate the process.

10. **Legal and human resource representatives** will likely have a unique perspective on safety issues.

The safety committee should represent a cross-section of your hospital. Committee members must actively participate in the business of the committee, such as performing site inspections or delivering reports on safety-related issues relevant to their particular disciplines. Members should help evaluate EH&S issues that you present to them. They should make decisions about how policies are developed and implemented.

If people sitting on the committee do not become involved, the committee will fail. You provide the leadership and expertise necessary to have a functional and successful safety program in the hospital. Yet you need to have a safety committee whose members can interpret the problems of the different units around the hospital—not only the safety problems but also the other issues that may confound or prevent the successful implementation of safety initiatives.

The safety committee members can help increase your effectiveness among the staff. Many times, the safety committee members are also department heads or supervisors. Ultimately, these individuals are responsible for safety in their unit or department. Their involvement and cooperation in the safety program is essential.

You may have to replace committee members if they do not participate or play an active role in the committee. Replacing committee members can be a difficult, even dangerous, task, potentially filled with political landmines. If a member needs to be replaced, speak with that individual privately. Find out whether he or she has a problem or why he or she isn't taking part. The individual may decide to resign from the committee before the chair is forced to ask him or her to leave.

Remember the safety committee members can help you spread the word about safety throughout your institution. They can also help you achieve the organization's EH&S goals and make sure employees and associates understand and comply with those goals. You cannot do it alone. So make sure that you have a committee that works with you.

Who is in charge of the safety committee?

There are several ways to determine who should lead the safety committee. In some hospitals, the safety director chairs the committee. Some organizations believe that since you are responsible for EH&S, you should head the committee that addresses these issues. This approach can work well. It reduces the number of steps in the reporting process.

On the other hand, when you chair the committee, there could be problems. You become responsible for the burdensome chore of organizing and running the committee. That's a sizable part-time job. It also means that you become exposed to the politics that are a part of running any organization-wide committee.

As an alternative, some organizations assign an administrative representative, such as a senior vice president, to head the safety committee. Having a member of the administration chair the committee demonstrates senior leaders' commitment to the safety effort.

It also frees you from many of the routine paperwork tasks associated with chairing the committee: organizing meetings, sending out notices, and keeping minutes and records. In addition, it helps buffer you from many of the political issues surrounding the operation of the committee.

Having an administrative representative in charge of the committee can work well. However, you will have to mentor the chair, since the chair typically does not have the background and skills required to interpret complex safety and environmental issues. Occasionally, having an administrative representative as chair of the safety committee can dilute the impact of the committee's reports to the CEO or governing body of the hospital, due to this lack of expertise in the areas of EH&S.

Some hospitals rotate the chair of the committee. These institutions allow a different member of the committee to assume the chair on an annual or biennial basis. In theory, each member of the committee will gain a greater appreciation of the challenges facing the committee and you. Of the three options, this creates the greatest risk of ineffectiveness because of the necessary start-up time, or learning curve, that each new committee chair will face at the beginning of his or her term.

This method also creates challenges for you. You must keep the committee focused and on schedule to effectively manage its workload. The time spent on educating and orienting a new chair every 12–24 months can be distracting for the committee and can mean delays in getting reports before the committee or delays in program implementation of new programs. Ensure that such delays do not have a negative impact on the progress of the safety program and the implementation of its components.

Where does the safety director fit in?

You play a pivotal role in the safety committee. Regardless of whether you chair the committee, you are involved in all aspects of its operations—from the inception of the committee and selection of the membership to the development of agendas and working schedules. You provide leadership, updates, and guidance about EH&S matters. This work begins in the committee. You help the committee meet its goals for ensuring that policies are developed and implemented in a timely fashion. The director and committee members review EH&S policies to see that they reflect all the standards of regulatory agencies, the hospital, and the JCAHO.

Develop a good working relationship with each member of the committee. They are counted on to help implement new policies and other EH&S initiatives in the hospital. They will be working on the front lines, making certain that these policies and procedures are practiced appropriately in their units and around the hospital. Rely on department heads, managers, and supervisors to ensure that safety policies and procedures are followed.

Most important to the EH&S effort are the employees themselves. Employees must hold themselves accountable for their own training. You are not the chief of the hospital's safety police. On a day-to-day basis, all members of the health care community must recognize you as the "go-to" person—an in-house expert who is available for information and guidance in interpreting safety policies and implementing safety practices.

Participate in other hospital committees that affect employee, patient, and neighborhood EH&S. Some committees may deal with such matters as hazardous waste handling and disposal, materials handling, latex glove use, or construction issues, to name a few. By taking part in these committees, you can share opinions that help facilitate a safe and healthful environment.

Educate hospital staff. Take part in the process of educating and training new employees in such areas as fire safety, emergency response, and the safe handling and disposal of chemicals.

Your role is sometimes difficult. While you are usually a part of the administration, you cannot play the role of administrator only. While you are an employee, you cannot play the part of an employee only. And while you represent the needs of EH&S, you must be a leader, not a crusader.

You must be credible to be effective, evenhanded and impartial. At times, you must be a neutral arbiter of safety and environmental issues that provide for the betterment of the hospital workers and their neighbors. Similarly, you must be open to new ideas and new approaches to the resolution of problems.

What about subcommittees?

In most hospitals, the safety committee consists of subcommittees with various responsibilities that work to support the goals of the committee. Subcommittees might be designed to inspect various portions of the hospital. Others might review various types of incidents or track quality improvement initiatives in various departments.

One or more subcommittees should be in charge of inspecting inpatient and common areas, such as corridors and offices, maintenance shops, laboratories, housekeeping storage areas, and materials handling and storage areas, to name a few. The larger the hospital, the more complex the facility, the more diversified the committees.

For those institutions that operate in several different locations that are separated by large distances, it might be necessary to have subcommittees that are responsible for routinely visiting and inspecting each of these off-site locations.

In addition, a health care institution may have on-site laboratories where hazardous materials are used and stored and where hazardous wastes are generated. In this case, you might want to establish a subcommittee responsible for inspecting laboratories.

In each case, the subcommittee should have a chair or leader responsible for organizing and leading that group. The safety committee chair typically appoints the subcommittee members. The leader needs to maintain records and present the results of inspections to the safety committee. Take part in each of the subcommittees. Of course, the greater the number of subcommittees, the more spread out you will become. If the structure warrants it, you might need an assistant.

Do not try to use the members of the safety subcommittees as safety policemen. Use subcommittee members to assist you and the departments they represent to achieve better safety performance. Use these members to build a safety team that can work together with you in a cooperative fashion to achieve goals that you alone could never reach.

Safety subcommittee members can work within their departments to help organize the employees and assign responsibilities within the departments for safety-related tasks. You can then utilize these assigned employees and the others who work with them to discuss the safety objectives of the unit, the issues that they are working on, whether they have been successful in their efforts, and what new approaches they might use to improve their safety efforts. In this way, two-way communication can be developed and fostered between the employees working on safety issues in the department and you. Of course, throughout this entire process, department supervisors and managers are kept informed and involved.

Managing the safety committee

The chair of the safety committee is most often the formal manager of the committee. The chair will bring the viewpoint of senior administration to the committee so that members understand the administration's position as they fulfill their duties.

Build consensus and set the tone for the safety committee so that its members support your goals for achieving a safe and healthful work environment.

By way of constant education and discussion, you keep committee members informed and up to date about what safety problems are present in the hospital, what environmental health and safety issues are looming on the horizon, and what steps the organization needs to take to comply with regulatory requirements. Keep the committee members informed about any evolving or critical issues that could have a negative impact on the hospital and develop good working relationships with committee members. Your credibility will enable you to lead the committee and use it effectively.

Getting the most out of the committee and its members

The safety committee and its members need to be active participants in the safety program. Work closely with committee members, motivating and educating them to help him create a culture of EH&S. Of course, this will not work 100% of the time. However, once the members of the safety committee and subcommittees begin to work cooperatively with you, the safety program becomes a shared responsibility. There is a synergistic effect. Not just one person is preaching the gospel of safety. Many people are. They are working toward the same end sharing goals and objectives that can be realized across the institution.

What to look out for

The safety committee may run into problems. Sometimes buy-in and cooperation are scarce. There are pitfalls that come with the job. Here are a few common problems that you might face, along with suggestions to deal with them:

Problem: Everyone expects you to perform all the committee's functions—that is, all inspections, reports, etc. In other words, the safety committee needs motivation in order to perform.

Solution: Educate committee members, department heads, and the committee chair about safety. The program works only when responsibility is shared . Stress that you cannot implement safety for the entire organization; you can, however, facilitate EH&S practices with the assistance of hospital staff.

Problem: People within the organization do not want to alter their behavior and attitudes about safety and environmental issues.

Solution: Exercise both patience and finesse, while at the same time educating the naysayers so that they can move forward and try new techniques. For example, safety professionals often find that employees have done a particular job in a certain way for their entire career. A new analysis of the data and injury information shows that a change in the procedure can significantly reduce the number of employee injuries. Use your wits, skill, and experience to convince both safety committee members and hospital employees that a change in the way they do things will not take any longer but will reduce injuries. One example is elimination of the old tradition of mouth-pipetting chemicals in the laboratory. New and improved techniques for lifting and moving patients to reduce repeat stress trauma are another.

Problem: Politics can be very disruptive. Some individuals or groups might not perceive EH&S policies and procedures as being in the best interest of their departments. One example might be the institution of policies and procedures for use during construction to ensure that patient and employee safety is maintained. While everyone agrees with the sentiment of the policies, some might think that such policies are too costly and/or impede the rapid completion of work.

Solution: You need to work to develop a good relationship with those responsible for construction. Demonstrate how these policies are good not only for the patients and employees, but also for the construction workers and the project. Not only does the implementation of these policies reduce liability for the hospital, it can help reduce risk of harm to patients during construction.

Problem: Regardless of how congenial you are, personality clashes can come into play and hinder progress of the program.

Solution: Be a team builder, a team player, and a team leader.

Problem: You are only an administrator in disguise.

Solution: Walk a fine line between manager and employee. You cannot decide disputes among management and employees, should be the arbiter and facilitator of EH&S issues only, must be impartial and fair, and must be willing to represent management when management is right about safety issues and to represent the employees when they are correct.

Problem: On some occasions you will have to deliver bad news about a problem or situation that exists in the hospital. The problem may even involve outside agencies, such as OSHA or the EPA. The messenger can sometimes be the target or outlet for the anger felt by others on the safety committee, senior administration, or others within the facility.

Solution: Approach the issue calmly and firmly, and offer a rational solution. Finger-pointing or assigning blame should not be a part of the discussion. Discussions surrounding the matter at hand should be about solving the current problem and preventing similar ones in the future. Fact-finding reviews should take place after the immediate problem has been resolved.

When the safety structure already exists

An EH&S program may already exist at your facility. An existing safety committee may have been in place for some time. The members already may have concepts of what to expect from the safety program and from a safety director. Entering such a situation can be difficult. Preconceived notions are held not only by committee members but also by the safety professional.

Accordingly, you need to take some time to get to know the committee members and learn about the other safety players. Further, you need to assess what expectations these members of the safety team bring with them. Be careful to establish your credibility with the safety committee members.

While all this does not have to be done in a day, a week, or a month, it should be done in a relatively short time. Otherwise, you might not be capable of making changes in the program—how it operates and how the committee members interact and behave. You will bring new perspectives and new ideas to the hospital. Whether your ideas flourish or are snuffed out depends on how you establish relationships on the first day. Cooperation must accompany knowledge.

Chapter 3

The Manual

You are going to be responsible for writing policies and procedures for the safety program. You will also need to either assemble or revise the safety manual. Not only are these unenviable, time-consuming tasks, they also are often very challenging. However, they are necessary for many different reasons.

The safety manual acts as a guidebook for the safety program, the safety committee, and your hospital. It is the blueprint for what is expected of employees with regard to safety matters, and it defines all the safety-related requirements that employees are expected to follow. A written manual ends all doubt—although not necessarily all discussion—about the safety program. The manual helps employees interpret and identify the essential rules for EH&S.

Of course, the safety manual can serve other purposes. Use it as a means of showing OSHA and EPA regulators or JCAHO surveyors how the organization communicates important safety issues. It will also display how the organization has interpreted, managed, and implemented safety regulations.

A word of caution: The safety manual is only as good as the documentation that backs it up. In other words, if the manual indicates that all employees are trained upon hire in a specific regulation—hazard communication, for instance—you must be able to demonstrate this. Be ready to produce written records proving that you have implemented the program as stated in the safety manual. Have at hand training material and records of attendance. If the manual states that all employees who handle infectious waste are educated upon hire and annually thereafter, you need immediate access to written records proving that the organization has met the commitment.

Writing policies and procedures

Writing, in and of itself, can seem daunting. Just the thought of it frightens most people. Writing and assembling a safety manual only adds to the anxiety. The regulations and requirements that you must assemble and include are numerous. And you can organize the information in a variety of ways. Foremost, remember that the manual must reflect the activities and demands of your hospital.

Purchasing or copying prepackaged, commercial hospital safety manuals in which the buyer fills in the blanks with the facility's name might ease the burden of writing, but it won't produce a manual that fits your specific needs. It is harder, but in the long run better and more efficient, to create a manual that meets and matches your organization's unique conditions. Ultimately, the safety director and hospital administration and you are accountable for the contents of the manual and how it is circulated and implemented.

When preparing a manual, you likely will focus on the regulations that are driving the development of policies and procedures. However, keep in mind that the force behind those policies and procedures should be the health and safety of employees, patients, and neighbors. Writing a manual for compliance purposes only will lead to failure.

There are a number of different ways that safety directors write and assemble safety manuals. One approach many safety directors have adopted, especially during the past few years, has been to assemble the safety manual in accordance with the JCAHO requirements. As a result, several hospitals have changed the safety manual to the EC manual. The topics covered in such a manual consist of the seven standards within the EC section of the JCAHO's requirements:

- Safety
- Life safety
- Security
- Hazardous materials and waste
- Emergency preparedness
- Medical equipment
- Utility systems

Other safety directors organize the safety manual by topic or area of concern, such as fire safety, emergency preparedness, electrical safety, laboratory safety, respiratory protection, equipment safety, etc. Manuals organized this way include the seven areas covered by the Joint Commission. However, manuals organized in this manner place less emphasis on the JCAHO requirements alone and take into consideration the organization's priority, which is to establish a safety program that is based on the unique needs and requirements of the hospital itself. Of course, many institutions—especially those starting a safety program from scratch—use the JCAHO requirements as a starting point for program development.

Carefully consider the amount of information included in the manual. Initially, you might plan to assemble a manual that includes all the organization's policies and procedures and every pertinent reference and requirement. This method, while complete, will often confuse many readers. The sheer volume of information might deter employees from routinely using the safety manual for reference. In this instance, often employees and staff clamor for a condensed version of the manual that is easier to use.

On the other hand, you might initially consider making the employee safety manual as concise as possible by including only the policies and procedures staff must follow. In this instance, all the regulatory references and details could be included in an appendix or a reference manual that is kept in an accessible location for anyone who cares to review it. Today, some hospitals maintain such reference materials electronically through an intranet.

Regardless of how you format your manual, consider all the important EH&S issues relevant to your health care facility. Moreover, prior to writing the manual, your safety committee must complete a hazard analysis and a survey of the entire hospital. These studies enable you to learn, firsthand, the issues that confront people who use and work in the facility.

Along with making sure your organization's policies and procedures meet the Joint Commission standards, OSHA and the EPA requirements, and your local and state government regulations, don't forget local organizations, such as the fire department or the city's building code department. Often, the rules to follow are established by your local fire department, building department, etc., or, as they are often referred to, the authority having jurisdiction.

When in doubt about which requirement to follow in a particular area, it usually is safe to adhere to the most stringent requirement. Your organization might discover potential EH&S problems that are not covered by any rule, regulation, or standard. Here are some examples:

- Should the hospital allow pets to visit their sick owners? Some psychologists say that such visits help patients heal faster. However, is it good for the hospital, other patients, or visitors?

- Should the hospital limit cell phone use? Although it may be necessary to restrict cell phone use in locations with a high volume of telemetry equipment, what about the rest of the hospital?

- Are plants a problem? Should the hospital restrict plants from some areas of the patient population?

- What kinds of plans must the hospital have in place to deal with visitors who come to see a patient infected with TB?

- Can patients bring in computers for use in their rooms?

Writing the safety manual requires some discipline and organization on your part. Assemble all the pertinent rules and regulations. Collect all the organization's existing safety-related policies and procedures. Next, adopt a manual style that is easy to understand and logical. The following is a checklist of EH&S organizations that have reference material related to policy development:

- OSHA
- EPA
- State and local ordinances
- Fire department codes
- National Fire Protection Association
- American Society of Heating, Refrigeration, and Air Conditioning Engineers guidance documents
- American Institute of Architects guidance documents
- CDC
- The JCAHO
- National Institute of Occupational Safety and Health
- Department of Transportation
- American Industrial Hygiene Association
- American Conference of Governmental Industrial Hygienists
- American Society of Safety Engineers
- Policies and procedures that already exist in your facility

Getting safety policies and procedures approved

Typically, policies, procedures, rules, and regulations that serve as the basis for your safety program need approval of the safety committee and senior management before you can include them in the safety manual. In order to have the elements of the manual go through in a relatively smooth fashion, you once again need to manage the members of the safety committee. You must discuss with them the various policies you are considering. Educate them about the regulatory source of each rule and why it needs to be included in the safety manual.

In some instances, a member of the safety committee might be able to lend his or her expertise to some safety manual matters, such as electrical equipment or utilities. Involve your internal experts whenever you can; ask them to draft the initial version of the policy or procedure. You can then act as the editor or as an assistant, helping them to prepare the document and ensuring that they use the appropriate language to meet hospital standards or regulatory requirements.

Involving safety committee members as part of the team needed to prepare and enact safety policies and procedures helps ease the way for approval of these policies by the safety committee and senior administrators. Senior administrators may not know the regulatory requirements or the policies for managing utility systems or handling hazardous waste, for example. They rely on you, the safety director, and the members of the safety committee to provide them with the correct information.

Once the safety committee has worked with you and has approved the contents of the safety manual, senior administrators typically feel that they are supporting the correct decisions when they adopt the policies and procedures contained in the manual.

CHAPTER 3

Keeping ahead of the game

Members of your organization cannot ignore the safety manual until it is time
to update it once every three years for the Joint Commission's survey.
Hospitals in today's health care environment face a virtual onslaught of new
regulatory requirements. As indicated in Chapter 1, hospitals have come under
a great deal of scrutiny by almost every regulatory agency imaginable.
Changes in thought and philosophy about how to protect patients and visitors, workers and staff, and neighbors of the facility have been occurring on an
almost monthly basis. These changes come from regulatory agencies, concerned citizens, activist groups, and advisory organizations like the JCAHO.

Often, these ideas are incorporated into new regulatory requirements in such
a short time that it is almost impossible to keep up. Think about the changing
requirements that have occurred regarding mercury-containing chemicals in
hospitals, or indoor air quality, or the use of latex gloves, or respirator use by
health care providers when tending to patients infected with TB.

You will need to monitor these changes continuously. Think ahead and plan in
a proactive fashion about how the information in newly uncovered hazards or
evolving safety issues may affect the institution and its neighbors. The FDA has
looked at the potential hazards that might be contained in the plastics used to
deliver intravenous fluids to babies. Scientists are starting to speak out about
the presence of persistent biological toxins in manufactured goods and their
effects on the endocrine system.

Certainly, you do not want to enact a policy or procedure before you have a
firm understanding of the issue and its meaning to patients and staff. However,

THE HOSPITAL SAFETY DIRECTOR'S HANDBOOK, SECOND EDITION

as this information becomes available, and as the discussion of these topics becomes more common both in the hospital and in the general population, you need to be in position to address these issues effectively and intelligently. Have educational materials ready and ideas about how and where these problems will affect EH&S in the hospital. Hopefully, by the time an issue is fully formulated through scientific discussion and debate, you will have educated the safety committee and senior management and will be prepared to make changes and enact new policies and procedures.

Educating staff

No safety program or set of policies and procedures can be effective until two things happen:

- Organization members understand the requirements
- They adopt these requirements into their daily practice

Any successful safety program depends on employee education. Engaging workers while teaching, and explaining policies and procedures to them are extremely important. The primary resource for this employee education is the safety manual that you've written. Employees should know, through education and training, that when they need answers they can refer to the safety manual and that this resource is the standard for everyone who works in the facility.

It's important to point out that the policies and procedures were not developed in a vacuum, but were created as a result of the correlation of regulatory requirements with the hospital's everyday practices. Be sure to communicate to employees that the safety manual was written not to make their jobs more difficult or cumbersome, but to make their workplace safer and healthier.

You might experience difficulty getting people to attend safety training sessions. For one thing, people do not often find safety education very exciting. And some believe that safety is merely a matter of exercising common sense. In fact, hospital safety is a marriage of a wide variety of scientific disciplines, as exhibited in fire safety, for example. The key to safety education is to strike a balance between what employees need to know to perform their work safely and what they should know to move to the next level of safety awareness.

Strong safety training session attendance is often quite simple. Typically, it is listed as a requirement for employees to complete as they start work, receive their annual review, or, in the case of nurses, renew their license certification. Having a good working relationship with supervisors and the support of senior hospital administration makes the enforcement of the rules for annual safety training for employees easier for the safety director.

Training needs to contain more than rote recitation of the policies and the requirements. A brief discussion of the background and reasons for the development of the policies helps people remember why they must follow them. Looking at fire safety as an example, people in hospitals need to understand whether they can safely evacuate to the next fire compartment, or zone of refuge, during a fire or leave the building immediately. In either situation, explaining the logic for either action helps people understand what they should do and why they should do it. It helps them incorporate the correct behavior into their decision-making.

Finally, it is important to establish safety training as a normal part of the worker's job assignment. This begins on the first day of work at new employee orientation. Some organizations provide all the safety training an employee needs during that first orientation session. Most, however, break up the safety training and use the new employee orientation as an introduction that guides employees to the various training sessions they must attend. Some sessions, such as fire safety, may be universal. Other sessions, such as use of TB respirators, hazard communication, and electrical safety may target a particular audience.

EH&S training and education provide the framework for a successful and functional safety program. Once the safety manual is written, approved, and distributed, ensure that the policies and procedures contained in the manual are incorporated into the culture of the hospital.

Chapter 4

Budgeting for Safety

Creating a budget is an essential part of your job. Even if the EH&S budget composes only a segment of a larger departmental budget, it is important to make sure that there is a place where the expenditures that you will need to make will be accounted for financially.

In some instances, the safety budget may actually be divided among several departments. For example, money for safety education and training might fall under human resources, while the money for environmental compliance might be found in the engineering budget.

Either way, the budget you create needs to take into account all of the direct and indirect costs of the safety program and its operation. Often the organization for which you work will set out fiscal guidelines and financial goals for the entire hospital for the upcoming year.

Regardless of the fiscal climate, EH&S will need to compete with other support service departments, such as security, environmental services, and materials handling. Sometimes safety needs will even have to vie with the cost of capital expenditures requested by patient care operations. There are, after all, only so many dollars to go around.

Your EH&S budget might start out as a large, all-encompassing financial needs assessment, but then be honed down to a finer level based on budgetary constraints placed on safety and other departments by the hospital's administration. As in the case of any other business unit, lack of funding can often lead to lack of success in your mission.

Getting the budgetary needs right is good for you and good for the hospital. Demonstrate that you understand the fiscal responsibilities that have been placed upon you by the hospital, while still assuring that employees, visitors, patients, and your neighbors are protected through the safety department.

Sizing up needs

As you begin to develop a budget, take into account the needs of the safety program. Some budgets may be all-inclusive, encompassing both operational and capital cost requests. Others may divide up the budget, with operational costs being funded at one time during the year and requests for capital expenditures, such as large pieces of equipment, being funded under a separate request at a different time of the year. Regardless of how this is handled at your hospital, you need to assess both sets of needs on an ongoing basis.

The first consideration in the budget should be safety department staffing needs. What safety director has ever felt that their staffing levels are perfect as is? One way of approaching the evaluation of staffing needs is as follows:

   1. List all routine tasks performed by the safety department—include both technical and clerical tasks.

2. Apply the time that it takes to perform each task.

3. Add these times up and divide the total by 2,080. You will recognize the number 2,080 as the number of hours worked by one person during one year (40 hours per week, 52 weeks per year). You might wish to add up the times under the various categories you have defined, for example: inspections, monitoring, waste collection and disposal, clerical, JCAHO preparation, etc.

Don't forget to add some additional, but reasonable, time for emergencies or unexpected events. Are employees paid by the hour or are they on salary? Is overtime pay going to be needed?

Along with staffing needs are the costs of education and training for the staff to ensure that they maintain their skill level. Most hospitals today will pay for a course or a training program per year per employee. What about conferences and seminars? Most hospitals today do not pay for organizational memberships for individuals or for certification maintenance.

Using this information, you can then determine

- staffing needs for EH&S
- what kinds of positions you will need to define
- levels of training and education that staff will need (in smaller facilities, everyone may need to be a generalist and cross-training will be required)

The second consideration is equipment and supply needs. These requirements can be of several types:

1. Employee safety monitoring equipment and the materials that go with them, monitoring for exposure to chemicals such as formaldehyde, ethylene oxide, and waste anesthetic gases. Take into account the costs of equipment calibration, equipment maintenance and replacement, and the cost of an outside laboratory for sample analysis.

2. Environmental monitoring equipment—such as pH monitoring equipment for water waste stream effluents, or equipment to monitor indoor air quality parameters such as temperature, humidity, and carbon dioxide levels—may fall under the safety department's budget. Along with this equipment comes maintenance and replacement costs, and for pH equipment there may be also a need to purchase chemicals.

3. Personal protective equipment used by members of the safety department, including respirators, gloves, and Tyvek suits, as well as equipment used by others in the hospital, including TB respirators and face shields for nursing and goggles for laboratory personnel.

The safety department's budget will also include various operational costs, such as those for chemical waste disposal, including permits, storage containers and safety cabinets, the actual waste disposal costs, and spill control and cleanup equipment; education and training materials and supplies, including books, videos, library costs, overhead projectors, slide projection fees, computers, educational programs, and office supplies such as paper, pens and pencils, computer supplies, mail, telephones, fax machines, and pagers.

Note that the fees for chemical waste disposal often provide fertile ground for debate among department heads and administrators. This debate usually revolves around who should pay these costs: the hospital or the individual departments. Although there is no definitive answer, most believe that relegating these costs to the individual departments can often lead to problems.

The problem that people most often worry about is the improper disposal of waste chemicals by some, often well-meaning employees who are trying to reduce the department of some of its budgetary overhead. The best solution, followed by the majority of institutions, is to pay for these costs centrally.

The previous lists are only suggestions to help you try to identify all the materials, supplies, and equipment that you might wish to account for as you begin to build your budget. Of course, the first time you do this will be the most taxing. However, it is important to remember that conditions and situations change from one year to the next.

Many hospitals that were able to add staff one year, for example, may be forced to cut back the next. Sometimes pressing needs crop up that should be addressed and resolved during the upcoming fiscal year, such as an unanticipated need to purchase additional monitoring equipment for conducting indoor air quality studies; or perhaps a study is needed to relocate the chemical waste storage room that was found to be unsafe following an inspection by the hospital's insurance company.

Accurate records and careful accounting will give you a better sense of how the budget needs to be changed or organized to confront the sudden needs and changing requirements of the hospital's safety program.

What size staff do you need?

There are probably a number of ways to determine the size of your safety department staff. There are some who recommend that one safety professional per 1,000 employees is a good number for low-hazard work environments. This number rises to two per 1,000 employees when there is a higher hazard level in the work environment.

However, if you refer back to the section on sizing up your needs in this chapter, you will find a method to help calculate the number of employees you will need in your department. This method helps put you on firm footing when it comes time to discuss staffing needs with your boss.

Safety department areas of expertise

The section on sizing up needs also discusses the need to define the types of positions that you will need in your department. Of course, while there are some common themes among safety departments, each one will differ, based on the nature of the operations at your facility. For example, if you work at an institution that is heavily invested in research, you will need to make sure that a member of your staff knows about chemical safety and hazardous waste handling. Ergonomics is an important issue in safety today, and having a staff member who know about human engineering and workspace design may be helpful. And there is always a need for someone versed in life safety, including fire safety.

If your department is responsible for Joint Commission preparedness, hire an employee who has experience with JCAHO and in filling out the forms that go along with the preparation of the *Statement of Conditions.* You need employees who are versed in regulations, and, as safety director, you should be experienced in handling regulators and administrators, alike. Other areas of expertise should include an industrial hygienist to help perform monitoring for waste anesthetic gases and indoor air quality and an expert to teach respirator fitting for the tuberculosis program. Someone with a strong knowledge of general safety principles is also important. Consider a part-time employee who is trained in biosafety to help monitor the research or clinical laboratories in your facility. Of course, every safety department would like to have a trainer, but this is a luxury often unavailable to safety directors, especially in smaller facilities.

Identifying resources

The number-one source of money for the safety department budget is the hospital itself. However, in today's difficult economy, hospitals are under the gun to be operationally efficient, and the safety director may have to be creative in locating alternative funding sources for safety projects or department needs. Of course, this should be done with the full knowledge and cooperation of the administration and other involved departments.

For example, you might wish to have an ergonomics program in your hospital to help reduce back injuries to nursing personnel. Perhaps there is a public agency, or even a private one, that has funds available to pay for evaluation, education, and training. You might need to compete for the funding and assemble a team to administer and oversee the program. However, the advantages here are obvious because the cost of this program is underwritten not by the hospital but by an outside organization.

Perhaps there is a need to reduce the level of energy consumption in the hospital. Such a reduction would benefit both the community and the hospital by reducing the drain on the local energy supply while also reducing the cost of energy for the hospital.

Another environmental advantage would be a corresponding reduction in emissions from the power plant. Perhaps such a program, including the cost of items such as replacing light bulbs with more efficient bulbs, could be underwritten by a grant from the power company or a state or federal agency that has money available for these types of pilot projects.

In the end, when you are identifying the sources for money for your operation and your department, it might pay to be creative. Consider partnering with other groups in the hospital who, along with safety, may benefit from sharing the costs of projects and equipment with you. Also think of outside sources of money, including governmental and private agencies who may see an advantage in helping to support your efforts and those of the hospital for which you work.

Making the proposal

The safety department, like other hospital departments, usually needs to compete for funding on an annual basis. In order to be successful, the proposal has to be made so that administrators and budget officers can understand and appreciate its importance. The decision-makers also need to see the relevance. It is not enough just to say the safety office needs the money to avoid fines or comply with regulations. This type of request may get money, but probably only enough to cover the bare necessities.

The person presenting the budget must be able to clearly demonstrate what the requests represent and why they are essential. In addition, however, the presenter must be able to demonstrate not only the current value of these requests but also their long-term value.

Will the equipment you are asking for in this year's budget last a long time? Will it save on the cost of waste disposal, laboratory fees, or indoor air quality complaints? What will the value of a purchase made this year be in two years? In five years? How many employees can be trained with the educational materials you wish to purchase? How many injuries will be prevented? How much money will that save in workers' compensation costs?

When making the proposal for the safety department budget, put in extra effort, so that those who are evaluating your request see that the money you want to spend has value for now and for the future. Make them understand that the program that you represent has a value that, through investment in the budget, will become more valuable to the hospital community over time.

Preparing for the future

As indicated previously, a budget should not be stagnant. Nor should it be considered as having been written in stone. Budgets are for getting the job done. They are also a way to keep on track and prepare for the future. You should consider the budget to be an ongoing process, not one that is frozen in time each year.

First of all, it is more than likely that you will not get everything in your budget request that you want. So each year at budget time, revise and update your request, keeping in mind what you have and have not been able to achieve in past budgets. Use your previous budget requests as a building block for future budgets. Sometimes, you will be able to get only a portion of what you ask for or need. But that does not preclude you from putting together your needs over the course of a two-year time span. The key in this situation is to use what you have been given and demonstrate the successes you have had with those materials.

Also use the budget to trumpet successes that the safety department has achieved. For example, you might cite the reduction in worker injuries. Or you could show that by your budget process, you would achieve your goal of reduced chemical waste disposal costs over a three-year span, thus increasing the value of the budget dollar you received.

Budgetary successes and the way you use your budget builds the credibility of the program. These achievements also help foster a sense of assurance on the part of employees and administrators alike that you are doing the right thing with the safety program and the resources available to you.

Chapter 5

Surveillance Programs

The purpose of surveillance programs

Successful management of the safety program revolves, in large measure, around the maintenance of an adequate base of knowledge and information about what actually happens on a day-to-day basis inside your hospital with respect to EH&S practices. In fact, the acquisition of knowledge and information is so important that the JCAHO incorporated a section about information collection into the EC standards a few years ago. This information acquisition system is known as the Information Collection and Evaluation System (ICES).

There are many ways that a hospital or health care organization collects and analyzes data. One of the best, and most useful, methods is through surveillance rounds or inspections. In the case of surveillance rounds, the JCAHO has indicated what is needed, at least minimally, to have an adequate surveillance schedule. It has stated that surveillance rounds in patient care areas must be conducted at least two times per year.

Surveillance programs are important for reasons beyond meeting the JCAHO requirements. Surveillance programs give you the opportunity to meet face-to-face with department heads, supervisors, and employees on their turf, in their work areas. Use this time to listen to employees and to learn from them about every operation in the hospital. This will help you better understand the challenges each department and virtually each employee faces in trying to do his or her job. At the same time, the rounds provide you with an opportunity to build a relationship with staff while teaching them about the safety program in a more personal setting. It also gives you an opportunity to assist employees and the department to achieve safety goals by demonstrating support and providing direct help to those you are visiting.

Conducting surveillance rounds is also a chance for the safety director to market the safety program at the grassroots level. In other words, surveillance rounds help advance the culture of safety in the hospital through individual contact and relationship development.

A word of caution, however. You are not police. Surveillance rounds should not be used as a blunt instrument to force people into compliance or good safety practices. Rounds are another tool in the arsenal of safety management, as is managing by walking around.

Use the rounds to develop good working relationships with employees and their supervisors. You want them to talk to you and share their insights about safety and safety-related problems with you. You want people to know that you are concerned about their safety. You do not want to develop a mindset that says that employees should vanish or become invisible during the course of surveillance rounds.

Developing these attitudes and relationships will come in handy in the future. First, it will give you access to people when there are difficult decisions to be made or problems to be resolved. Good relationships and supportive employee attitudes will also pay off when inspectors from the various regulatory agencies such as OSHA or the fire department come to the hospital. These inspectors will want to question employees and speak with people randomly. They will want to get a sense of what is going on or delve into a problem and investigate it, if that is why they came in.

You will feel comfortable when this happens because you have worked hard to develop relationships and resolve safety issues with the very people being questioned.

How to establish effective surveillance programs

In order to be effective, surveillance programs need, first of all, to be initiated as a function of the safety committee. In that way, the surveillance rounds have the stamp of administrative approval and are established as a required function of an administrative arm of the hospital. Also, surveillance rounds need to be organized in a logical fashion on a routine basis with a given schedule and a time limit.

Some argue that to be effective, surveillance rounds need to be performed randomly and without advance warning. When surveillance rounds are conducted on a surprise, nonscheduled basis, you actually defeat the purpose of the rounds. Employees will feel surprised and angry that the safety program and its "police officers" are coming to catch them in the act of disobedience. They will disappear.

Real discussions about issues and concerns cannot take place, as surprise rounds typically evoke a confrontational attitude. The benefits mentioned previously about creating good relationships with employees and learning about the difficulties employees face in trying to get their work done disappear. Conversation is limited and real concerns do not emerge because people are concerned that someone is looking for a scapegoat to blame if there is a problem.

Not only should surveillance rounds be scheduled in advance, department heads or supervisors need to be involved in planning and scheduling rounds. Also, representatives from the department, both from the floor where the rounds will take place, as well as department administrators, such as a head nurse, should be involved in the surveillance rounds themselves, as well as in the evaluation of the findings and the reporting of the results. Of course, if problems are uncovered, the resolution of these problems should rest with the department personnel with your help or the assistance of someone else who may be qualified to assist in the resolution of the issue.

In addition, problems and concerns in hospitals, as we all know, are often the result of a combination of factors. For example, an indoor air quality problem may be your responsibility, but to fully resolve the issue, the head of engineering may also need to make sure that the air supply and exhaust system is working properly.

Surveillance rounds, then, should be a combined effort that encompasses many different departments who help support the mission of the patient care staff. The success of rounds carried out by an interactive and cooperative team is then made even more effective and time-efficient for the staff.

In addition, to be successful, surveillance rounds need a leader who is committed to the task at hand. You do not necessarily need to be the leader. In fact, it may be more useful to have the leader be a representative from the department where the surveillance is being conducted. So for patient care areas, the leader may be someone from nursing. Similarly, for the laboratory, someone from that department may take the lead.

Again, the most important element in having successful surveillance rounds is the development of an interactive and cooperative environment. Achieving observable and measurable results from the surveillance rounds is also essential to ensuring their ongoing success.

Keep records of what is found, and the findings must be reported in a timely fashion to the safety committee and the departments who have been reviewed. Also, the corrective actions necessary should be included in the report, as well as the time frame in which they are scheduled to occur. Results can then be compared from one surveillance inspection to the next, and changes can be noted.

Using this method, as mentioned previously, fits quite well with the ICES required by the JCAHO. The safety committee can track important elements. Sometimes such tracking and recording can lead to the discovery of a local problem that is readily resolved, such as a failure on the part of nursing staff to properly record the daily temperature of the refrigerator where drugs are stored.

At other times such tracking will uncover a problem that affects several different departments. For example, a problem with conducting practice fire safety drills may be occurring in several patient care units. Only after the surveillance rounds are conducted and the results recorded and compared does the problem become apparent. Once the problem emerges, then an investigation can be conducted to determine the underlying cause. A solution can then be devised.

Who should be on the team?

The team needs to be large enough to include an effective cross-section of support departments. Yet if the team is too large, the effectiveness and efficiency of the surveillance rounds could be impaired. Surveillance teams are typically a subcommittee of the larger safety committee. As people experienced in committee dynamics know, there are optimal sizes for committees to operate effectively. Typically, a committee or surveillance team should consist of only about six to eight people for optimal performance.

The team's composition needs to be dictated by what you are trying to accomplish. In fact, members of the team may vary from year to year, as a function of what information is collected, what is learned, and what issues surface.

Take into account, on a practical level, what departments compose the seven areas of the environment of care that might need to be included. Thus, safety, biomedical engineering, and security might be at the top of the list. Other representatives to consider might be housekeeping, maintenance, and infection control. In addition to these representatives, you will, in keeping with the concept of cooperation and inclusiveness, have a nursing or laboratory department representative join you, along with a representative of the area you are visiting.

What should you look for?

The idea of surveillance rounds is to perform a thorough, but not prolonged, inspection of an area and review of conditions. But surveillance rounds also provide an opportunity for the members of the team to speak with the employees and find out what is on their minds and their concerns. For example, is there a construction project being planned for the unit? Are staff worried about Interim Life Safety Measures during construction? Are they worried about control of noise and dust and the protection of patients from exposure to molds such as aspergillus? Do staff know what steps have been taken and will be taken to address these concerns?

Also review and discuss recordkeeping items, such as documentation of performance of practice fire drills, maintenance of logs of annual inservice training for staff, or the status of refrigerator temperature logs, at the time of surveillance rounds. If inservices are needed, use this time to schedule the safety training that the staff need.

Discuss any issues or problems that have been nagging at the personnel in the department. At this time, someone from the team may be assigned to assist the department in the resolution of the problem, as well as to follow up on the progress of that resolution and its aftermath.

Surveillance rounds are not complete unless they include a walk-through of the area. At that time, a visual inspection is made to review the condition of the physical plant, including cleanliness, the status of paint and trim on the walls, and the condition of the floors. The location and status of signs, such as evacuation or exit signs, can be evaluated. Although fire extinguishers are routinely checked, this visit provides the safety director an opportunity to see whether the inspection program is functioning properly.

In summary, surveillance rounds are meant to review all areas and aspects of the functioning of the unit. You and the surveillance team decide what to look for and what topics need to be probed further. These decisions, of course, are based on the knowledge and input of the personnel from the department and also on the historical record of past surveillance rounds.

Of course, if no history exists, then the time to start to build a historical record is now! Keeping track of issues and concerns, being active in the resolution of problems, contacting and interacting directly with employees will serve to help you and the safety committee get the most benefit from the surveillance rounds.

Do you need a checklist?

The question of whether a checklist should be used during surveillance rounds is a constant source of discussion. Safety professionals are always looking for the best checklist they can find. The checklist you develop for use in surveillance rounds should evolve from what you are trying to learn and what you are trying to teach staff as a result of the process.

The advantage of a checklist is that it provides consistency as you conduct surveillance rounds in different areas, and in the same location from one year to the next. While checklists are not the credo by which a safety director should live, it does help organize your work. It also helps those who participate in the surveillance rounds focus on the tasks and goals at hand. Checklists can also serve as training tools, as people become used to looking at the issues that you as safety director consider significant.

Take a look at Figure 5.1 on the next page for ideas of what to include in your checklist.

Figure 5.1

Surveillance Checklist

The following is an example of items that you might want to consider including in the checklist:

Safety issues
- Practice fire drills
- Fire extinguisher checks
- Safety education
    - Hazard communication training
    - Annual fire safety refresher
    - Respirator education and training
    - Needlestick prevention
    - Interim Life Safety Code preparation/education if construction is scheduled
    - Temperature charts for refrigerators/with proper temperatures
    - Proper storage of supplies in clean areas
    - Signs
    - Exit doors closed and stairwells free of storage and clutter
    - Oxygen cylinders properly secured

Environmental issues
- Housekeeping
    - Floors
    - Walls
    - Linens
    - High cleaning
    - Dusting
    - Trash disposal
    - Separation of contaminated objects (bloodborne pathogens)
- Indoor air quality complaints

Maintenance issues
- Walls

Figure 5.1

Surveillance Checklist (cont.)

- Ceilings
- Trim
- Walking surfaces
- Fire doors
- Exit signs
- Evacuation plans
- Condition of patient rooms and lounges
- Plumbing
- Elevators
- Stairwells clear and unobstructed
- Intercom systems and telephones

Biomedical engineering
- Up-to-date checks of equipment requiring annual review
- Daily checks of equipment where required
- Telemetry devices
- Presence of personal electrical devices that have not been approved

Security issues
- Valuables properly stored
- No unauthorized visitors on floor
- Pharmaceutical storage cabinets locked
- Employees wearing ID badges

Other
- Upcoming construction/renovation projects
- Problems not listed on check sheet

This list is not intended to be complete, but merely an example of a point at which to begin to develop a checklist.

Chapter 6

Committees and Communication

What are committees for?

There are many different views about committees and what purpose(s) they actually serve. Cynics believe that committees are a way of stalling and putting off decisions. Worse yet, some believe committees are a way of diverting decisions away from senior and mid-level administrators and managers to more junior people.

The truth is, however, that committees, when run properly and goal-directed, can be effective tools both for the hospital and for the safety director to accomplish difficult tasks. Committees can be the workhorses of a hospital, achieving important goals through a collaborative process.

The safety committee is a good example of this sort of activity. This committee has a specific framework and set of goals to accomplish, namely to be a responsible agent for oversight and direction of the hospital's EH&S program. Other committees could be formed to deal with issues such as use of latex gloves, adoption of a needleless device, or development of sound environmental policies for the hospital.

Of course, a variety of other committees that are established do not strictly involve EH&S. Yet many times, there are other committees throughout the institution where your input can be important. Two committees that fit this description include one that reviews the cleaning products used in the hospital and another that establishes specifications for the type of paint used in the facility. In each case, the resulting selection can have important effects on the health and safety of employees, visitors, and patients. Your input is needed in the discussions that take place in these committees.

For better or worse, hospitals today are more like other businesses than ever before and use committees both as an integral operating tool and as a management tool. In previous chapters, the advantage of hands-on, face-to-face contact with employees was noted, as well as the time-honored tradition of management by walking around. These direct interactions with employees and staff work very well and usually are very rewarding. However, the facts are that, many times, it is committees with broad authority or whose members have vested interests that make the decisions and determine the way that problems will be addressed or resolved.

It is important for you to be able to work effectively within the committee structure. Some committees are direct offshoots of the safety committee and some committees are formed from other administrative areas of the hospital. In either case, you should be invited to sit at the table in order to be heard on the issues that fall within your scope of expertise on environmental and safety matters.

Your views and professional input should be a part of the decision-making process. It is important to develop a reputation as a level-headed, clear thinker whose presence is welcomed, even sought after, and more important, whose input and opinions are valued and respected.

How to capitalize on committees

Committees, as stated previously, are tools. Use them to educate staff about safety and to incorporate safety policies as part of the solution to whatever problem the committee has been addressing. For example, what if you formed a committee to establish guidelines for conducting staff meetings in the hospital?

Suggest that as a part of the policy before every staff meeting, the chair must instruct attendees about the procedures to follow in the event of a fire alarm and the locations of the nearest exits. This is a simple two-minute exercise that reinforces fire safety and incorporates safety as a routine component of daily activity.

When EH&S concerns are included in committee decisions, everyone benefits. Staff have a better understanding that safety and safety procedures are practical and useful every day, not just at special times. By incorporating EH&S issues in all aspects of routine operation, the safety program helps change attitudes and behaviors, resulting in reduced employee injuries or exposures to hazardous situations, as well as increased practice in compliance and participation in safety activities. This way, you and the safety program gain an advantage and capitalize on the committee activities.

Establish effective communication with peers and leaders

In order to be effective, both as the safety director and as a committee member, it is important to learn how to effectively communicate with everyone, regardless of what position they hold or role they play in the hospital. Learning to be an effective communicator is an important part of any manager's job. Many managers, not just safety directors, never learn how to communicate properly or effectively. A number of self-help books have been written on the subject. Classes and workshops teach ways to communicate effectively.

When it comes to safety and environmental issues, employees and administrators throughout an organization often have different perspectives on an issue, whether it is the discharge of waste chemicals into the sanitary sewer or use of fume hoods for storage or evaporation of waste chemicals (an unacceptable practice).

As a committee member, establish yourself as a thinker who can clearly state a problem and recommend a solution. Demonstrate your ability to negotiate the difficult, sometimes thorny issues that arise with regard to EH&S matters.

One of the difficult safety issues that comes up will be convincing administrators that major renovations involving a commitment of thousands of dollars must be undertaken to resolve an indoor air quality problem. Similarly, it is sometimes necessary to convince employees that the indoor air quality problems that they have been experiencing do not require the expenditure of thousands of dollars and the initiation of major renovations.

Another difficult problem you may encounter is convincing employees to change their longstanding practices—practices that they may have been carrying out for years, and that have now been found to pose a hazard. Often, employees in the maintenance departments are reluctant to alter longstanding practices or to wear personal protective equipment when doing their work. Often, you'll hear "I've been doing it this way for years, and nothing has happened to me yet."

In the end, employees and administrators alike want to hear what you have to say about the issues. They want to hear the facts and have the issues placed before them in a calm, rational manner. People want to understand the concerns and, particularly managers, do not want to have a situation taken out of context or a problem blown out of proportion.

Do not put forth the issues with the worst-case scenario as an example—adding fuel to the fire. You will not be heard at all. Instead, you could develop a reputation as being a harbinger of doom, or someone who inspires fear by using inspections and fines as tactics to accomplish the job at hand. The result is usually disaster. For example, when work is to be performed that will involve the removal of asbestos from steam pipes in a patient care area, employees can often become very concerned.

Meet with the staff before the project begins, explain the procedures that will be taken to protect them from exposure, and assure them that no asbestos will escape from the area of removal.

But what about the case where all that happens and then employees come in to work the next morning only to find evidence that suggests that a breach of protocol and an accompanying leak of asbestos from the containment area did take place? You must direct the effort to find out quickly and efficiently what actually took place. If there was a breach, you must explain why it occurred, its extent, and its impact on employees in the area. People will look to you for guidance and honest answers.

Clearly state the issues and the pros and cons of the situation. Next, clearly state alternative solutions to the problem. Incidentally, that may mean that you need to say that, at the present time, you do not know all the alternatives. However, you must also state that you will conduct research and come back with a response. For example, as described in the asbestos example previously, you may not have the immediate answer to the question of whether a leak occurred and the size of the leak. Testing needs to be conducted.

Honestly tell people that the answers won't be available for several hours, but that in the meantime you are taking steps to ensure that they are protected. Explain what steps you have taken and why.

The key to communication is remaining clear and calm even when you are being harassed from both sides on an issue. Your role is to provide professional guidance and not to be argumentative or confrontational. Here are some other tips on communication:

- Make eye contact when speaking with individuals
- Listen, and try not to speak over or across others while they are speaking
- Allow people to express their views and air their opinions

Trying to stop this flow of communication and interactive dialogue only harms you and your reputation. In addition, when you do respond, never denigrate or show disdain for those who may not have all the facts or who may be misinterpreting the regulatory requirements. Certainly, arguing, raising your voice, or ignoring someone is not the way to go.

In addition to directly communicating with individuals, it is important to be able to communicate effectively in writing. Many people communicate best by e-mail. You must learn the skill of communicating in this way. Whether writing to a single individual or a group of people, be sure that you know e-mail etiquette. It is sometimes tempting to use e-mail as a way of speaking down to people. Write an e-mail the same way that you would address people if they were in front of you while you were speaking.

When politics rule the day

As has been discussed previously, hospitals are complex places. A wide variety of personalities, perspectives, and interests come together to operate and manage a hospital. Often, it is at the committee level that these divergent interests and viewpoints come together—and sometimes clash.

In some instances, contrary to what we may think, the resolution of safety or environmental concerns is not always clear-cut or black and white. Often, there is room for interpretation or, at the least, more than one way to reach the solution to a problem. Sometimes personal biases and egos can get in the way of finding a solution.

In some cases, a department head may feel put upon or threatened by the proposed resolution of a problem. That department head or manager may try to head off the resolution of the problem because the solution does not, for example, put him or her in a favorable light. For example, if the resolution of an indoor air quality problem is related to malfunctions of the HVAC system, you and the maintenance manager may have differing opinions both about the source of the problem and, ultimately, its resolution. Sometimes there is not enough information or evidence to support either person's point of view. The only resolution may come from a series of trials and errors.

Politics sometimes ends up being the key factor in the resolution of the problem, especially when there is no absolute regulatory guidance. As an example, injuries due to repeat stress trauma, particularly back, neck, and shoulder injuries, are known major causes of lost work time and workers' compensation payment in hospitals. Since the ergonomics regulations proposed in 2000 were never enacted, there is no regulatory requirement to take action, yet a conscientious safety director may propose some training and education to help reduce repeat stress trauma in the workplace.

Because head nurses may see this as an infringement on their territory, and because they may also see this new training and education effort in ergonomics—prevention of repeat stress trauma—as causing undue alarm among the nursing staff, the head nurses may band together to stop such a program from going forward. This appears to be a beneficial, relatively low-impact initiative, but it is steeped in politics.

The issue can lead to a clash between you and the head nurses—not because head nurses do not care about safety, but because it infringes on their area and may subject them to questions as to why steps have not been taken before. Politics ends up being the deciding factor in whether or not the program proceeds and is enacted.

What do you do when a situation becomes political? Don't be dramatic. Use the issue as a lesson from which you can learn for the future. Arguing or trying to make a stand on one political issue often has negative results that can adversely impact other aspects of the safety program. The negative results can range all the way from the development of a simple feud between the safety director and the other party to more dire consequences, such as dismissal of one party or the other, depending on who has the political power at the time of the event.

As part of your role as an effective communicator and leader, it is your job to move forward and develop an efficient, respected safety program and safety culture in your hospital. It is your job to demonstrate that your programming is not aimed at compromising any managers or department heads but is intended to assist them in improving the productivity of their departments by reducing injuries and illness and helping them improve the conditions for employees who work in the hospital.

As with all other jobs, some days everything goes right, and other days nothing goes right. The goal is to learn to deal with these small setbacks, while moving forward on the whole. Decisions made due to internal politics or the insecurity of some employees or managers are small setbacks that will be overcome by long-term goal setting and developing a reputation as a person whose purpose is to serve the best interests of the hospital and its employees.

Chapter 7

The Regulatory Agencies

Introduction

Health care is, if not the most regulated industry in America, certainly close to the top of the list. Until the mid-1980s, many regulatory agencies, OSHA and EPA foremost among them, did not pay particular attention to health care institutions. Hospitals were seen as safe havens doing good works and caring for the sick and elderly in our community. What possible harm could hospitals do to patients, employees, visitors, or neighbors?

Then, a change in attitude took place. America, with its heightened awareness of the potential safety and environmental hazards presented by manufacturing and construction and other heavy industries, began to suspect that hospitals might also be a hidden source of harm. The same questions that were raised about private industry—the chemicals used and stored, the way in which they were disposed, and the ways that employee and others were affected by exposure to accidental releases of these chemicals—were being asked about health care institutions.

Questions and concerns about the impact of hospitals on the environment and on public health came from a variety of sectors. Citizens and employee groups raised questions about the materials being used in hospitals to treat patients, and about their effects on employees and on the environment. Environmental groups such as the EPA and public health agencies asked about emissions from hospitals into public waters. Mercury and the use of products that contained mercury in hospitals that could affect fish also became concerns.

In the early 1990s, disposal of infectious waste raised a variety of questions about public health. Accompanying that concern was an awareness that incinerators used by hospitals to burn infectious wastes and the associated plastics may contribute to increased dioxin levels in the air. Effluents from the incinerators were also known to contain mercury and perhaps other metals, such as zinc. All these issues were accompanied by increasing awareness among nurses and other employees about indoor air quality problems, latex allergy reactions, and the potential for spread of bloodborne pathogens by needles or other contaminated materials.

Some of these questions were prompted by the emergence of new regulations and new reporting requirements, such as those requiring the reporting the presence of hazardous chemicals, accidental spills, and environmental releases of toxic materials into the air and water. Initially, these regulations were not directed at health care institutions. But they did raise awareness, and people began to ask questions: What was happening in hospitals, and how did these events compare with what was happening in industry?

Following closely on the heels of these questions were new concerns about the potential spread of devastating diseases to health care workers, such as

AIDS, hepatitis, and TB. Issues long present but often ignored by health care, such as indoor air quality complaints and workplace violence, were soon at the top of the list of health and safety concerns in hospitals.

The list of agencies regulating hospitals and nursing homes soon grew. OSHA and the EPA now cooperate with the Joint Commission by acknowledging one another's regulations and recognizing one another's existence as they tour a facility. The Nuclear Regulatory Commission looked at the use of radioisotopes and x-ray machines. Local organizations such as the fire department were joined by city and state inspection agencies. Not related to safety directly, but certainly related to patient care, were long lists of agencies, such as the Centers for Medicare & Medicaid Services, whose oversight on billing and financial matters could validate or overturn the findings of other agencies in areas related to patient care and patient safety.

Should your programs be designed with OSHA in mind?

Perhaps one of the earliest agencies to become aggressively involved in hospital safety was OSHA. As soon as the first regulations dealing with hazard communication became effective and their application to hospital settings was affirmed, OSHA became active in inspecting and reviewing hospital employee safety issues. OSHA's position in hospital safety was reinforced by the leading agency in ensuring that hospitals were safe places to work and safe places to be a patient, the JCAHO.

The JCAHO quickly adapted its long list of safety standards and safety requirements to reflect the OSHA standards and, later, the environmental safety requirements of the EPA. In fact, there are now written memoranda of understanding among these three groups that if an inspector from one group uncovers a concern in another's area of responsibility he or she will share that finding. So, if an OSHA inspector finds a violation of an EPA requirement, he or she will share that finding both with the EPA and with the Joint Commission, thus possibly causing an unpleasant and embarrassing experience for the hospital.

Today, the JCAHO's safety requirements are consolidated and reflected by the seven sections of the EC requirements that all health care facilities must comply with in order to be accredited by that organization. Such accreditation means that hospitals are eligible for Medicare and Medicaid reimbursement. With all the changes that have occurred over the past decade in hospital economics and health care financing, every hospital wants to succeed in its routine inspections and reaccreditation visits from the JCAHO. One way of attempting to ensure compliance has been to change the way that safety manuals and safety programs are designed and written. Many hospitals have taken the lead from the Joint Commission and rewritten their safety manuals to reflect the seven topics cited in the JCAHO's EC standards:

- Safety
- Security
- Hazardous materials and waste management
- Emergency preparedness
- Life safety
- Medical equipment (biomedical engineering)
- Utility systems

Although it is important to consider each of these areas in the design of the safety program and to include them in the safety manual, it is not necessary to design your safety manual as a compliance guide for the JCAHO environment of care standards. Similarly, while it is important to keep the OSHA worker safety and EPA environmental compliance requirements in mind as you design your safety program and develop your safety manual, you do not need to make your safety manual look like a miniature JCAHO compliance document or a code of federal regulations guidebook.

Your safety manual and the safety program itself need to represent the hospital for which you work and its philosophy on patient care and EH&S. In other words, a hospital needs to be involved and proactive in protecting its employees from hazards in the workplace.

It also needs to consider its effects on the environment—the materials and byproducts of its treatment programs. What types of wastes is it sending out to the local waters? Are emissions from the hospital and its laboratories having an impact on the ambient air around the hospital? Is the hospital contributing to levels of pollutants such as oxides of nitrogen? These issues need to be considered and addressed in safety plans and in the design and development of hospital systems.

The safety manual should reflect the regulations and compliance guidelines that need to be followed, but in the context of the values that the hospital, its administration, and executive board hold.

A safety manual should reflect the needs of the safety program and describe the goals the program is attempting to achieve and the rules and policies that are in place to reach those goals. Merely following the regulatory requirements set forth by any of the agencies mentioned will probably ensure compliance for your facility. However, remember that the requirements spelled out by each of these agencies reflect only the minimal level of actions and activities that need to be carried out to be in compliance.

If you want your safety program to excel, it must transcend those minimal requirements and go beyond the mere basic compliance requirements. In short, your safety manual needs to take the EPA, OSHA, and JCAHO regulations and guidance documents into account, but it does not need to be a regurgitation of the information in the same format.

The changing face of OSHA

OSHA has inserted itself more and more over the past few years into the health care workplace. Regulations covering bloodborne pathogens, laboratory safety, and needlestick protection lead the list. As discussed in Chapter 6 of this handbook, OSHA fell short of enacting ergonomics legislation in 2000, but in a changing approach, set forth nonmandatory guidelines for ergonomics that would still be enforced by targeted inspections and citations under the "general duty clause.[1]"

In 2002, and after more than 30 years with the same format, OSHA updated and amended the reporting requirements for fatalities, injuries, and illnesses required under 29CFR 1904. Among the casualties was the familiar OSHA 200 form. A new series of 300 forms was created. The log for maintaining injury and illness records is now known as the 300 log. In addition, OSHA created a 300-A log to serve as the summary form for annual reporting of the information recorded on the 300 log. The incident reporting form is known as

---

[1] Section 5(a)(1) of the OSH Act

the OSHA 301 form, although if your facility has its own form that captures the same details as the 301, you may continue to use that.

Changes in the basic requirements of what needs to be recorded were not altered. In other words, all work-related injuries, illnesses, and fatalities must still be recorded. Record an illness or injury if it involves the following criteria: "Death, days away from work, restricted work or transfer to another job as a result of the injury or illness, medical treatment (beyond first aid), loss of consciousness, and significant injury or illness diagnosed by a physician or other health care professional."

This last point means that when a professional health care provider makes a diagnosis of significant injury or illness, regardless of any of the other criteria being present or not, the event becomes recordable.

In 2002, OSHA added criteria to the recordkeeping requirements. Included among these were needlesticks and sharps injuries, TB, and situations that required removal of employees from their job because of medical reasons. Incidents of hearing loss will also need to be recorded beginning in 2004. However, the issue of musculoskeletal injuries (ergonomics) still remains a cantankerous issue, and had originally been included on the OSHA 300 log, but in the form's final revision, officials removed it.

An important, and often difficult decision, even if you are experienced, is determining whether an injury or illness is recordable. OSHA has attempted to cut down some of the confusion by making the requirements for recordability the same for both injuries and illnesses, a departure from the past. Thus, an injury or illness must be considered work related if an event or exposure in the work environment caused or contributed to the resulting condition or aggravated a preexisting injury or illness. To determine whether an injury or illness is recordable, OSHA provides the following decision tree[2]:

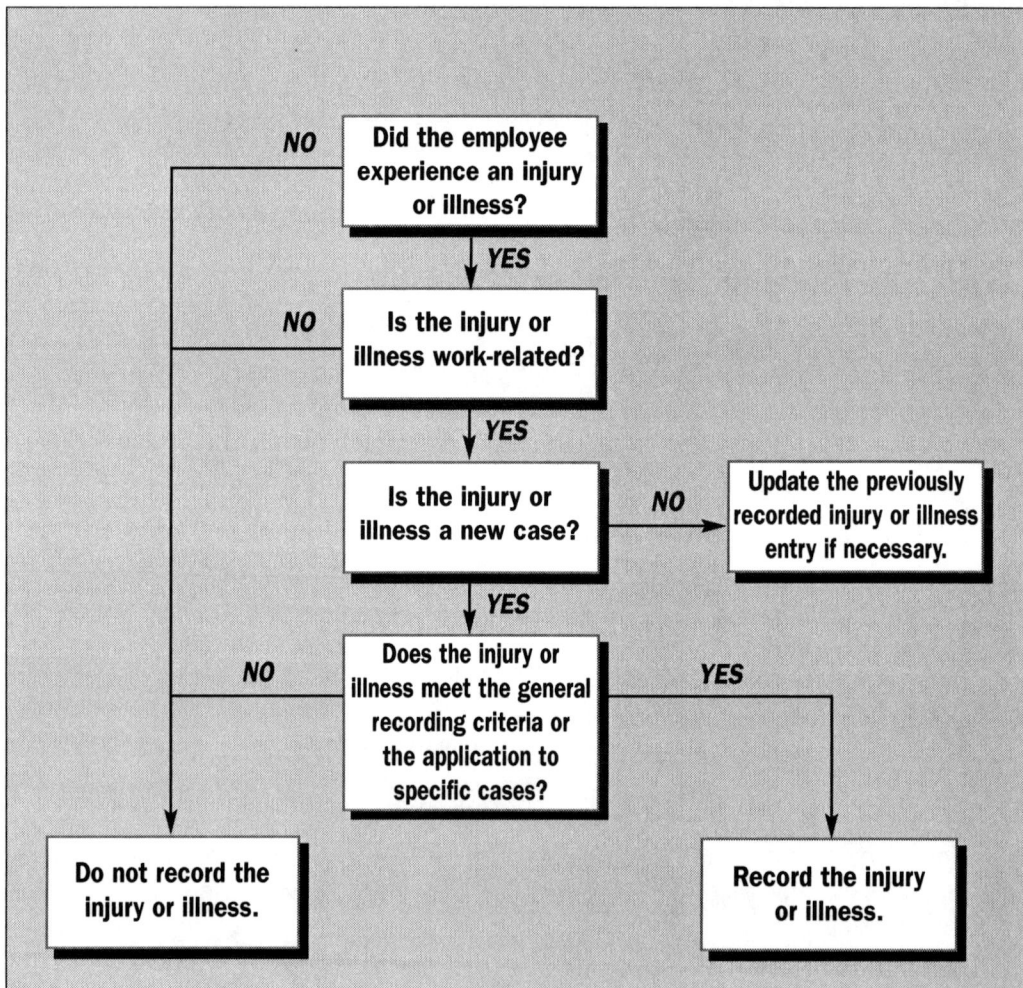

2 29 CFR 1904.4 (b) (2)

There are, however, certain exceptions to the requirement that injuries or illnesses occurring in the workplace need to be recorded as work related. The following are some examples of injuries and illnesses that should not be recorded on the OSHA 300 log[3]:

- At the time of the injury or illness, the employee was present in the work environment as a member of the general public rather than as an employee.

- The injury or illness involves signs or symptoms that surface at work but result solely from a non-work-related event or exposure that occurs outside the work environment.

- The injury or illness results solely from voluntary participation in a wellness program or in a medical, fitness, or recreational activity such as blood donation, physical examination, flu shot, exercise class, racquetball, or baseball.

- The injury or illness is solely the result of an employee eating, drinking, or preparing food or drink for personal consumption (whether bought on the employer's premises or brought in). For example, if the employee is injured by choking on a sandwich while in the employer's establishment, the case would not be considered work-related

(**Note:** If the employee is made ill by ingesting food contaminated by workplace contaminants, such as lead, or gets food poisoning from food supplied by the employer, the case would be considered work-related.)

[3] 29 CFR 1904.5 (b)(2)

- The injury or illness is solely the result of an employee performing personal tasks (unrelated to his or her employment) at the establishment outside of the employee's assigned working hours.

- The injury or illness is solely the result of personal grooming, self-medication for a non-work-related condition, or is intentionally self-inflicted.

- The injury or illness is caused by a motor vehicle accident and occurs on a company parking lot or company access road while the employee is commuting to or from work.

- The illness is the common cold or flu (Note: contagious diseases such as TB, brucellosis, hepatitis A, or plague are considered work-related if the employee is infected at work).

- The illness is a mental illness. Mental illness will not be considered work-related unless the employee voluntarily provides the employer with an opinion from a physician or other licensed health care professional with appropriate training and experience (psychiatrist, psychologist, psychiatric nurse practitioner, etc.) stating that the employee has a mental illness that is work-related.

There are, of course, some other areas that lend themselves to confusion in making the determination about whether to record the injury or illness. Perhaps foremost among these items is the definition of medical treatment. For the purposes of 29 CFR 1904, medical treatment means the management and care of a patient to combat disease or disorder. Medical treatment does not include visits to a physician or other licensed health care professional solely for observation or counseling; the performance of diagnostic procedures, such as x-rays and blood tests, including the administration of prescription medications used solely for diagnostic purposes (e.g., eye drops to dilate pupils); or first aid.

29CFR 1904(7) defines first aid as using a nonprescription medication at nonprescription strength (for medications available in both prescription and nonprescription form as recommended by a physician or other licensed health care professional). The use of a nonprescription medication at prescription strength is considered medical treatment for recordkeeping purposes.

There are several treatments that at first glance may appear to be medical treatment, but which are actually considered first aid under the recordkeeping requirements. Some examples include the administration of tetanus immunizations, which are first aid. Yet, other immunizations, such as hepatitis B vaccine or rabies vaccine, are considered medical treatment. Other types of treatments that are considered first aid include cleaning, flushing, or soaking wounds on the surface of the skin; using bandages, gauze pads, butterfly bandages; and hot or cold therapy. The list goes on but is conveniently spelled out in the pages of the regulation.

The following is a side-by-side comparison of the old injury and illness standard versus the new standard[4]:

4 From Directive # CPL 2-0.131, *Recordkeeping Policies and Procedures Manual*, 1/1/02.

Old Rule	New Rule
Forms §1904.29	
OSHA 200 - Log and Summary OSHA 101 - Supplemental Record	OSHA 300 - Log OSHA 300A - Summary OSHA 301 - Incident Report
Work-Related §1904.5	
Any aggravation of a pre-existing condition by a workplace event or exposure makes the case work-related	**Significant** aggravation of a pre-existing condition by a workplace event or exposure makes the case work-related
Exceptions to presumption of work relationship: 1) Member of the general public 2) Symptoms arising on premises totally due to outside factors 3) Parking lot/Recreational facility	Exceptions to presumption of work relationship: 1) Member of the general public 2) Symptoms arising on premises totally due to outside factors 3) Voluntary participation in wellness program 4) Eating, drinking and preparing one's own food 5) Personal tasks outside working hours 6) Personal grooming, self-medication, self infliction 7) Motor vehicle accident in parking lot/access road during commute 8) Cold or flu 9) Mental illness unless employee voluntarily presents a medical opinion stating that the employee has a metal illness that is work-related.
New Case §1904.6	
New event or exposure, new case	Aggravation of a case where signs or symptoms have not resolved is a continuation of the original case
30 day rule for CTDs	No such criteria
General Recording Criteria §1904.7	
All work-related illnesses are recordable	Work-related illnesses are recordable if they meet the general recording criteria
Restricted work activity occurs if the employee: 1) Cannot work a full shift 2) Cannot perform all of his or her normal job duties, defined as any duty he or she would be expected to do throughout the calendar year.	Restricted work activity occurs if the employee: 1) Cannot work a full shift 2) Cannot perform all of his or her routine job functions, defined as any duty he or she regularly performs at least once a week
Restricted work activity limited to the day of injury makes case recordable	Restricted work activity limited to the day of injury does not make case recordable
Day counts: Count workdays No cap on count	Day Counts: Count Calendar days 180 day cap on count
Medical treatment does not include: 1) Visits to MD for observation only	Medical treatment does not include: 1) Visits to MD for observation and counseling only

2) Diagnostic procedures 3) First aid	2) Diagnostic procedures (including administration of prescription medication for diagnostic purposes) 3) First aid
First Aid list in Bluebook was a list of examples and not comprehensive	First Aid list in regulation is comprehensive. Any other procedure is medical treatment.
2 doses prescription med - Medical Treatment (MT) Any dosage of OTC med - First Aid (FA) 2 or more hot/cold treatments - MT Drilling a nail - MT Butterfly bandage/Steri-Strip - MT	1 dose prescription med - MT OTC med at prescription strength - MT Any number of hot/cold treatments - FA Drilling a nail - FA Butterfly bandage/Steri-Strip - FA
Non-minor injuries recordable: 1) fractures 2) 2nd and 3rd degree burns	Significant diagnosed injury or illness recordable: 1) fracture 2) punctured ear drum 3) cancer 4) chronic irreversible disease
Specific disorders	
Hearing loss - Federal enforcement for 25dB shift in hearing from original baseline	Hearing loss - From 1/1/02 until 12/31/02 record shift in hearing averaging 25dB or more from the employee's original baseline
Needlesticks and 'sharps injuries' - Record only if case results in med treatment, days away, days restricted or sero-conversion	Needlesticks and 'sharps injuries' - Record all needlesticks and injuries that result from sharps potentially contaminated with another persons blood or other potentially infectious material
Medical removal under provisions of other OSHA standards - all medical removal cases recordable	Medical removal under provisions of other OSHA standards - all medical removal cases recordable
TB - Positive skin test recordable when known workplace exposure to active TB disease. Presumption of work relationship in 5 industries	TB - Positive skin test recordable when known workplace exposure to active TB disease. No presumption of work relationship in any industry
Other issues	
Must enter the employees name on all cases	Must enter 'Privacy Cases' rather than the employee's name, and keep a separate list of the case number and corresponding names
Access - employee access to entire log, including names; No access to supplementary form (OSHA 101)	Access - employee and authorized representative access to entire log, including names; Employee access to individual's Incident Report (OSHA 301); Authorized Representative access to portion of all OSHA 301s
Fatality reporting - Report all work-related fatalities to OSHA	Fatality reporting - do not need to report fatalities resulting from motor vehicle accident on public street or highway that do not occur in construction zone
Certification - the employer, or the employee who supervised the preparation of the Log and Summary, can certify the annual summary	Certification - company executive must certify annual summary
Posting - post annual summary during month of February	Posting - Post annual summary from Feb 1 to April 30
No such requirement	You must inform each employee how he or she is to report an injury or illness

Bloodborne pathogens and needlesticks

In addition to the changes noted previously, there are other changes with respect to needlestick protection. OSHA adopted the Bloodborne Pathogens Standard (29 CFR 1910.1030) in 1991 in order to protect workers exposed to bloodborne diseases. OSHA revised the standard in 2001. The revisions were made in response to passage of the Needlestick Safety and Prevention Act (Pub.L. 106-430,66 Fed. Reg. 5317). This act reflected the results of 10 years of experience showing a major source of exposure to bloodborne pathogens resulted from needlesticks and contaminated sharps.

The Needlestick Safety and Prevention Act directed OSHA to revise the Bloodborne Pathogen Standard. The changes established clear requirements that employers identify and use safer and more effective medical devices in order to reduce injuries from needles and sharps. In addition, the act included two new terms in the standard and modification of one existing term. The two new terms added were:

A. Sharps with Engineered Sharps Injury Protection

1. This is defined as a " non-needle sharp or needle device used for withdrawing body fluids, accessing a vein or artery, or administering medications or other fluids with a built-in safety feature or mechanism that effectively reduces the risk of an exposure incident."

2. This term covers a broad range of devices, including syringes with a sliding sheath that shields the attached needle after use needles that retract into the syringe after use shielded or retracting catheters intravenous

medication delivery systems that use a catheter port with a needle housed in a protective covering

B. Needless Systems

1. This is defined as a device that does not use needles for:
    a. the collection of body fluids or withdrawal of body fluids after initial venous or arterial access is established
    b. the administration of medications or fluids
    c. any other procedures involving the potential for occupational exposure to blood borne pathogens due to percutaneous injuries from contaminated sharps.

2. Examples of these devices are:

    a. intravenous medication systems that administer medications or fluids through a catheter port using non-needle connections.
    b. jet injection systems that deliver liquid medication beneath the skin or through muscle.

The term "engineering controls" was modified because the original Bloodborne Pathogen Standard was not specific with respect to the applicability of various engineering controls in the health care setting. In the original version of the standard, engineering controls were meant to refer to devices "that isolate or remove a hazard from the workplace, such as sharps disposal containers and self-sheathing needles."

See Figures 7.1 and 7.2 for examples of a bloodborne pathogen survey and a form to record employee participation in selection of safer needle devices.

The revised standard now specifies what is meant by effective engineering controls. Such controls now refer to "safer medical devices, such as sharps with engineered sharps injury protection and needleless systems" that must be used where feasible.

New additions were also made to the exposure control plan. These changes require employers to take into account any changes in technology that will lead to the elimination or reduction of exposure to bloodborne pathogens. Employee input is a key element in the selection of safer medical devices for use in patient care. It is anticipated that the devices selected will not compromise employee or patient safety, and that such devices will reduce the likelihood that an exposure incident involving a contaminated sharp will occur.

In addition, all safer medical devices that have been identified and considered for use in the facility need to be included in the documentation that employers must keep to show that a decision process has been used to advance the protection of employees from needlestick and sharps injuries. As part of the process, the employer must also document the methods used to evaluate all such devices and maintain records for justification of selection of the safer devices.

Although the selection of safer devices to prevent sharps and needlestick injuries often falls under the purview of the infection control professional, you need to stay current on such matters, if not totally involved in the process, since this is a key element in protecting employees from injury and illness in the health care workplace. And, you most likely will perform or assist in the investigation of needlestick incidents and who will most likely be responsible for the recordkeeping aspects of the incident.

Workplace violence

One more area that has received a great deal of attention is workplace violence. Although OSHA has no specific regulation covering workplace violence, the agency has issued recommendations to protect employees from violent acts. Workplace violence is the third leading cause of workplace fatalities in the United States, and health care workers are approximately four times more susceptible to violent attacks, assaults, and physical threats than other workers in private industry.

Workplace violence prevention is an important part of the health and safety program of any institution, and the JCAHO also requires it, although the development and oversight of the program typically falls under security. As you may be responsible for security, you must develop a workplace violence prevention program. Such a program should include administration involvement and support, an analysis of the workplace to look for potential or existing hazards where violence can occur, implementation of work practices and engineering controls (such as glass windows and locking devices) in areas that present a hazard, health and safety training to make staff aware of the program, and the potential dangers and ways to protect themselves. Finally, the program should also include recordkeeping for injury and illness reporting and an evaluation program to ensure that it is effective and updated, as needed.

Figure 7.1

Bloodborne Pathogen Survey: Job Classification and Tasks at Risk

Name of Institution_____

Date _____

Department _____

Location (several locations may exist; one form per location)_____

Name of Person conducting Survey_____

A. List of tasks/job classifications where exposure to sharps may occur

_____

_____

_____

_____

_____

_____

B. List of tasks/job classifications where exposure to blood or other contaminated material may occur

_____

_____

_____

_____

_____

_____

Figure 7.1

Bloodborne Pathogen Survey: Job Classification and Tasks at Risk (cont.)

C. Classification of tasks/job classification by severity of risk (from high to low)

_____

_____

_____

_____

_____

_____

_____

D. Evaluation and comments:_____

_____

_____

_____

_____

_____

_____

E. Recommendations: _____

_____

_____

_____

_____

_____

Figure 7.2

Employee Participation in Selection of Safer Needle Devices

Name of Hospital_____

Department: _____

Team Leader: _____

Meeting Dates (maintain a separate sheet for each meeting):_____

Names of participants and job titles:

_____

_____

_____

_____

_____

_____

List of all devices considered:

_____

_____

_____

_____

_____

_____

Figure 7.2

Employee Participation in Selection of Safer Needle Devices (cont.)

Methods and criteria used to evaluate each device_____
_____
_____

Justification for selection of devices to be added: _____
_____
_____
_____
_____
_____
_____

Writing to the regulators

One of your biggest challenges will be communicating with regulatory agencies, particularly in a written letter of response as a result of a complaint made against the hospital by an employee or some other individual. You are also responsible for the written response made to a regulatory agency following an investigation or an inspection. Most safety directors, hospital administrators, and other professionals who are experienced in dealing with regulatory agencies know that writing to these agencies can be tricky and laced with pitfalls. The first rule in dealing with any regulator is: Be honest.

But dealing with regulators is somewhat like testifying in court. You need to be clear about what is being asked of you and, once you are clear, answer only the question that you have been asked. This may sound a little dubious, as though you are trying to evade something, but it's not.

Once you make assumptions and answer questions or parts of questions that have not been clearly asked, you could be leaving yourself and the hospital you represent open for criticism or, worse yet, some type of action by the regulatory agency you are dealing with. Therefore, be honest in all your responses, but make sure you are responding only to the question being asked.

Most often, a written response to a regulator such as OSHA or the EPA comes either as the result of an employee complaint or as the result of an inspection. When responding to such a matter, remember that the key is to collect all the facts. Sometimes you will have only a few days to do this and to respond.

Typically, when an employee makes a complaint to OSHA, you will receive a phone call informing you that a complaint has been made and the nature of the complaint. This will be followed by a written document detailing the articles of the complaint. In this situation, you will usually have only four or five days to gather as much information as possible to write a response. The format of the response should look something like the following:

1. A restatement of the complaint and each of its separate specific items.

2. A summary of the facts that you have gathered concerning the complaint. Remember, it is neither fruitful nor important to determine who made the complaint or identify the real motivation for the complaint.

3. A statement about what, if any, steps have been taken to address the complaint immediately.

4. A list of actions, such as monitoring, sampling, and/or hiring a consultant, that will be taken to address the problem in the short term. This is particularly important if you have found a problem exists that you need to acquire more data on.

5. A timeline for getting back the results and instituting any changes, repairs, etc., that will need to be done as a result of the sampling and monitoring.

6. Include photographs, monitoring results, etc., that you already possess.

7. Provide a timeline for future activity and include additional documentation of results when it becomes available.

It is important that you respond quickly and efficiently to any letters of complaint from regulatory agencies. First, a rapid response will help avoid an on-site inspection by the agency. Also, a diligent response will help you establish a good image and positive reputation with the agency. Good will can go a long way in helping to work through problems as they arise in the future because the agency representatives soon learn who is truly responsive and concerned about EH&S.

Establishing a good working relationship with representatives of the various regulatory agencies will not prevent problems, but it will help you better understand the inspector's expectations when a problem does come up.

What to do when the inspector arrives

Unfortunately, not every response to a regulatory agency is done by mail. If OSHA, for example, receives a signed, written complaint rather than a telephone call, the inspector will show up at the front door of the facility to conduct an inspection. A few years ago, the EPA conducted surprise inspections of research laboratories at universities and hospitals to determine compliance with hazardous waste regulations.

When the inspectors show up at the door, you have the right to refuse them entry. However, as they will return with both a court order and a bad attitude. Let them in, ask to see some identification, and notify the proper people in your administrative chain of command that the inspector is on-site.

Have a contingency plan already in place with a team of personnel who will accompany the inspector. That team might include you, an administrator, and a member of the safety committee who represents the department or area where the alleged violation occurred. It is also important to keep in mind that there are some items the inspector will always look at: your OSHA injury and illness log and, typically, some other required programs, such as your hazard communication program.

When the inspector arrives, you will want to find out the nature of the complaint and the location of the concern. You will want to lead the inspector to that location, once your contingency team participants show up, as quickly and in as short a route as possible. Understand, however, that the inspector inspects any location he or she wishes. Also, if the inspector observes an infraction of any type, even one unrelated to the issue that brings him or her to your facility, he or she can issue a citation for that infraction.

During the course of the inspection itself, the inspector will interview employees in private. If your facility belongs to a union/unions, the employee does have the right to have a union steward present during the interview. On the other hand, the employee is not required to speak with the inspector or answer questions.

All these facts demonstrate very clearly why it is important to have good relationships with employees so that they will speak with you or register their complaints before they get to the point of calling OSHA or EPA. Some employees will still prefer to report their complaints anonymously.

Many hospitals have set up just such a system, with a 24-hour telephone answering service that allows employees to report their concerns without identifying themselves.

The key here, of course, is to follow up and investigate the complaints and, if a complaint has a basis in fact, to resolve it. Trying to discover who made the complaint is unproductive and a waste of time.

Chapter 8

The Joint Commission

Introduction

The Joint Commission has been mentioned throughout this book. The purpose of the discussion presented in this section is not to provide you with yet another compilation of the JCAHO guidelines. Instead, this section is designed to provide you with some practical viewpoints on the types of activities and the level of involvement that you need to have in order to be prepared for a successful JCAHO inspection.

The Joint Commission preparation process in days gone by was a triennial event. Yes, the safety program and its elements were in place every day, but only in the face of an impending inspection did you bring out the JCAHO manuals, dust them off, and review them. Today, that has changed.

For one thing, the JCAHO visits are still trienniel events, but random, unannounced surveys can occur from nine to 30 months after the last accreditation survey. About 5% of accredited organizations are surveyed this way. You need continuous monitoring of programming efforts and their effects. To address this concern, many hospitals have started ongoing programs that are designed to involve the key JCAHO planners and implementers within the hospital in JCAHO-related issues oversight. The projects and teams routinely meet to review the procedures and record keeping required by the JCAHO.

During these ongoing meetings, key players review and update the SOC to ensure that these documents accurately reflect the conditions in the hospital as they exist at the time of the JCAHO visit. If, for example, the hospital does not have sprinkler systems as part of the fire protection system, then this needs to be shown in the SOC. This document then allows the JCAHO planners to provide a schedule and a plan of action for addressing this deficiency by installing a sprinkler system. The plan can also show the time frame and actual plan for adding the system over the next so many months.

The SOC also provides the JCAHO planners the opportunity of keeping abreast of any changes that have been made in the physical plant that will need to be addressed in the SOC. They also oversee and review the progress made on any required changes or upgrades that were instituted in response to the last JCAHO visit. In addition, if any Type I recommendations were made during the last inspection, this group ensures that corrections have been made and that they are appropriately reported to the Joint Commission.

Yes, JCAHO inspections have led hospitals to a state of ongoing preparation and continuous oversight to eliminate that last-minute rush to get things done. You will be the central figure, leading the group through its paces as they update and prepare for the review of the EC. (See Figure 8.1 for an example of progress improvement goals.)

What is the EC?

As every health care safety professional knows, the essential hospital support functions, including safety, are now rolled up into one component that the JCAHO has termed the EC. The EC is made up of several different subsections, namely safety, security, hazardous materials and waste management, emergency preparedness, life safety, medical equipment (biomedical engineering), and utility systems.

In a large number of hospitals, many of these functions, including security, fall directly under your oversight. If there are exceptions, they would most typically be medical equipment and utility systems. Yet even these two areas frequently require your input. For example, when an accident occurs involving medical equipment, you become a party to the investigation. The extent to which you might become involved in medical equipment failure problems and investigations is highly variable, and in some way is a reflection of the quality of the medical management program and the level of vigilance associated with that program.

Failures of medical equipment, such as beds, can injure patients. In some cases, you may actually uncover a medical device problem during the course of your routine activities. For example, while monitoring the operating rooms for levels of waste anesthetic gases, you may find a higher than expected level of the gas in the room air. Upon investigation, you may find that the medical device used to supply the nitrous oxide to the patient is defective and needs to be repaired or replaced. Similarly, the oversight and maintenance of utility systems involve patient and employee safety elements, such as routine generator testing or the assurance of water supplies during disasters.

Figure 8.1

Progress Improvement Goals

Below are some examples of the progress improvement goals that might be established in the safety, security, emergency preparedness, life safety, hazardous materials and waste, utilities management, and medical equipment areas:

- **Facility safety:**
  - Increased attendance at fire safety training
  - Faster response to emergency calls
  - Improved management of the information collection and evaluation system
  - Development of new safety education modules

- **Security:**
  - Reduced number of thefts
  - Increased passage of patrolling officers
  - Improvement in investigative reports
  - More involvement with local police

- **Emergency preparedness:**
  - Increased participation in community-wide practice drills
  - Improved evaluation of unscheduled events
  - Development of new programming for potential terrorist attacks
  - Improved methods of communication within the hospital during a disaster

- **Life safety:**
  - Better participation in practice fire drills
  - Improved tracking of performance of fire alarm signals
  - Reduction in the number of false alarms
  - Improved method of tracking fire extinguisher inspections

Figure 8.1

Progress Improvement Goals (cont.)

- **Hazardous materials and waste:**
  - Improved auditing techniques for chemical tracking
  - Assurance that all departments have up-to-date material safety data sheets (MSDSs) for the chemicals they use
  - Improved methods for locating hazardous materials on site, such as asbestos
  - Assurance that monitoring for waste anesthetic gases (WAGS) is conducted on a routine basis and that the results are reported to staff and discussed with them in a timely fashion.

- **Utilities management:**
  - Testing of all emergency generators on full load monthly
  - Tracking of all system failures and follow-up remediation
  - Scheduling routine maintenance for all utility equipment
  - A set schedule for replacement of aging equipment

- **Medical equipment:**
  - Calibration of all defibrillators daily
  - Proper labeling of all equipment and tagging with routine calibration dates
  - A set schedule for routine maintenance of anesthesia equipment
  - Testing the function of telemetry equipment on a routine basis

When the JCAHO rolled out the EC standards, new requirements were soon added to strengthen them. Each component within the EC standards had to have an up-to-date management plan prepared for it. In addition, performance improvement goals needed to be set in each area.

This also meant that hospitals had to develop a way of clearly demonstrating what those goals were and what relevance each one had to the program under discussion. In addition, methods had to be designed to measure improvement within those target areas over time.

When the JCAHO visit takes place, the inspector will ask to see each management plan. He or she will also ask for a demonstration of the performance improvement for at least one of the goals that have been established. It is important, therefore, to keep the management plans current, along with the indicators and measures of the goals and progress that have been achieved.

What you need to know

First and foremost, know that you are the person on whom most employees and administrators will depend to provide leadership in the hospital's JCAHO preparation efforts. Also know that the JCAHO guidelines as provided in the EC section of the JCAHO manual are not necessarily the last word in health and safety programming for the employees of the hospital.

These guidelines are, rather, the basic starting point for a health and safety program, as are the OSHA requirements in 29 CFR 1910. Yet the JCAHO guidelines in conjunction with the OSHA requirements are important to the hospital and to its leadership, as they provide the key elements for maintaining Joint

Commission certification and, ultimately, ensure that federal Medicare and Medicaid funds continue to flow into the hospital coffers.

As a result, understand how to work effectively with employees throughout the hospital. Be able to assist employees to understand the safety program and best comply with it. Help staff understand programming as it relates to the JCAHO guidelines.

Be aware of issues that present the biggest challenges to hospital employees. In particular, know what workplace issues could most prevent employees from complying with good safety practices. Figure out the facility and identify environmental problems that exist there.

Environmental problems may include a wide variety of issues. Some of the more common items seen are indoor air quality complaints about poor air circulation, odor, and temperature. On some occasions, noise or vibration problems negatively affect patient care and employee performance. In some cases, there are rare and uncommon environmental problems.

Of course, you then need to work to help resolve these issues—not just for the JCAHO but for the improvement of conditions on an ongoing basis. In addition, understand the stresses that employees experience. Although these stresses are present on a routine basis, they become amplified when employees know that the Joint Commission inspectors are coming and will focus, to a large extent, on them as they are quizzed about a variety of issues, including their role in safety.

Employees often feel the tension and the stress projected by supervisors, administrators, and others, including you, as you are trying to create a scenario for an excellent JCAHO visit. Employees and others can sometimes lose their sense of focus, not to mention their sense of humor, in an effort to perform well and demonstrate their level of excellence to the JCAHO surveyor.

At all times, everyone must keep in mind the real purpose of his or her job in the hospital—caring for patients, not pleasing outside surveyors. Ensure that employees remember what they have already learned and practiced about the various elements of the safety program, whether it's fire safety, emergency preparedness, or hazardous waste.

Finally, you need to know your role when the JCAHO inspector comes. You can help make the inspection process go more smoothly for the hospital and for employees. Ensure that many questions are answered before the inspector actually tours the facility and interviews employees. This can be accomplished during the opening document review session by having a well-thought-out presentation about the safety program, its achievements, and the measurement of the performance goals. Offer information during the review session that answers key questions before the inspector needs to ask them; the entire JCAHO inspection and review process will go more smoothly.

Assessing the safety program

Typically, the safety program gets a thorough review when everyone knows that the JCAHO triennial review is coming. In truth, such an assessment of the program should occur more often—at least annually, at the time when you need to submit a report on the past year's achievements and stumbling blocks to the safety committee. An honest review of the safety program and the department's activities will help avoid many of the problems that often arise when the Joint Commission's visit is only a few months away and there is a realization that some elements of the program have been neglected.

Rushing to collect data or to repair the damages of oversight or, worse yet, neglect, of various program elements is, to say the least, a poor reflection of the safety program, you, and the safety committee. It is also the best way to end up with a bad Joint Commission visit and at least one Type I recommendation.

When reviewing the safety program and performing an assessment, the best place to start is to look at your safety manual. An appraisal needs to be made of each element of the program and of the goals that have been set for the year. A discussion always ensues during a safety program assessment about benchmarking—comparing your program to others of similar size at similar hospitals. This comparison is a good idea, and it works well for those programs that are already operating at a high level of performance.

Before you reach that point, however, you need to benchmark your program against the internal landmarks that you and the safety committee deem important and appropriate. In addition, there is often a great deal of discussion about what yardsticks to use as a basis for measuring the success of the program. One element that invariably comes up is the injury and illness rate as reported on the annual OSHA report form. This is probably not the best base for comparison, however, as those rates are generally subject to many variables that are not really under the control of the safety director, including the actual level of reporting of injuries and illnesses. Other pertinent benchmarks

need to be selected, such as monitoring of employee exposure to waste anesthetic gases, proper understanding of material safety data sheets, or use of
appropriate personal protective equipment.

Finally, as mentioned previously, many hospitals have changed the way that they
prepare for Joint Commission inspections. Rather than preparing eight to 12
months before the planned visit, these hospitals have initiated programs that
maintain readiness by continually reviewing elements of compliance and ensuring that program changes and facility improvements are monitored and docu-
mented.

A number of programs, such as monitoring employee exposures to hazardous
chemicals or waste anesthetic gases, should be ongoing and not be initiated
only when the JCAHO visit is looming on the horizon. Safety education and
training, such as hazard communication training, should be a part of the routine mix of safety programming. This ongoing monitoring along with data collection during surveillance rounds can go a long way in helping to assess the
status of the safety program and the attainment of its goals.

Consultants

Hospitals may wish to use consultants as a means of assessing the safety
program or to help them prepare for the Joint Commission inspection.
Consultants can be an effective way of bringing in third-party reviewers
with different perspectives to help evaluate the current status of safety
programming or the hospital's position with regard to its EC program.

Consultants can be effective and useful if used properly. Perhaps one of the
most important things to consider when choosing a consultant is reviewing his

or her experience. There are many consultants, for example, whose only experience is as third-party observers: They have never actually managed a safety program, worked in a hospital, or undergone a Joint Commission review or OSHA inspection. Make sure the consultant you hire can prove his or her claims and have actually performed tasks that have me the needs of other programs.

Consultants may make recommendations and work with you to assess the program and ensure that it is in compliance with the various regulations; however, they are not ultimately responsible for the success or failure of the program. It is not the consultant's job to ensure that safety requirements are met, be it training or monitoring exposures to hazardous materials or reporting spills in a timely fashion to the proper authorities. It is your job. Therefore, all consultants need to be managed.

Remember that consultants, no matter how experienced or highly qualified, work for whoever hired them, whether a safety director or an administrator. So use consultants when appropriate, but use them wisely.

Chapter 9

Bioterrorism: The New Challenge

Weapons of mass destruction and bioterrorism, or fears of them, have invaded every aspect of our lives. Since the terrorist attacks of September 11, 2001, all of us have been bombarded—virtually on a daily basis—with information about the potentially damaging effects of a bioterrorist attack.

You must now deal with the prospect of mass casualties exposed to chemical, biological, or radiological materials entering your facility's emergency room at almost any time of day or night.

You and your staff need to be prepared to treat patients who may have been exposed to those harmful materials.

Understand the types of materials your facility could encounter in a bioterrorist event. Become familiar with methods of treating patients, particularly those who have not first been seen by emergency response personnel or not been decontaminated. Establish procedures to protect staff from exposure and contamination when they evaluate and treat victims.

It is interesting to note that for the past several years, the EPA has required hospitals with emergency rooms and that treat casualty victims to use personal protective equipment when dealing with contaminated patients. In recent years, the JCAHO has weighed in on this requirement as part of the hazardous materials section of its regulations. In doing so, the JCAHO cites and virtually extends the OSHA requirements under 29 CFR1910,120(q) for treatment of those who have been exposed to hazardous chemicals.

The newest requirements for emergency response capabilities in the face of potential terrorist attacks using chemical or biological weapons significantly affects hospital emergency preparedness requirements. September 11, 2001, pushed hospitals and medical staff to learn more about decontamination procedures and the use of personal protective equipment.

In fact, in 2003, medical schools and hospitals all over the country instituted educational programs to help physicians become better prepared to deal with and treat patients exposed to or contaminated by chemical and biological weapons. These programs have also improved physicians' knowledge of protective equipment, including respirators.

For example, Vanderbilt University Medical Center in Tennessee has established the National Center for Emergency Preparedness. The program's goal is to become a model for other schools and medical centers around the nation in ways to best educate and train health professionals and emergency response personnel in the prevention, detection, and response to weapons of mass destruction.

In 1972, the United States and many other countries signed the "Convention on the Prohibition of the Development, Production and Stockpiling of Bacteriological (Biological) and Toxic Weapons and on Their Destruction," commonly called the "Biological Weapons Convention." Yet, this treaty has been, for all intents and purposes, ignored. It has had very little deterrent value among many nations.

Emergence of anthrax

Anthrax thus far has been the only material successfully used as a biological agent in the United States following September 11. Government officials and the public expressed shock that unknown persons contaminated envelopes with anthrax in several U.S. locations in 2001. Several of those people exposed to the contaminated envelopes became ill; six died.

Historically, anthrax, or wool sorters disease, was relegated primarily to farmers and people who came in contact with the fur or hides of contaminated animals. It was unimaginable before 2001 that anthrax could be "weaponized," or produced in such a way as to maintain both its ability to remain airborne and keep its viability. The fact that the latter was accomplished while sending contaminated envelopes through the U.S. Postal Service was even more astonishing—and informative.

Based on the unexpected success of the anthrax attacks, federal agencies identified and put under scrutiny other biological materials that could be used as weapons. Foremost among the biological materials now under consideration is smallpox, which is caused by the variola virus. It is now believed that smallpox, like anthrax, can be effectively used as a biological terrorist weapon.

Unlike anthrax, which requires the victim to have direct contact with the bacterial spores, smallpox can be readily spread among individuals by direct contact with an infected person or by handling contaminated items, such as blankets or bedding.

Smallpox is a very serious, often fatal, disease that has no cure or available treatment. Historically, smallpox infection results in the death of about 30% of those infected. Vaccination can help prevent or reduce the effects of smallpox infection.

However, there is a great deal of controversy and concern over possible side effects that may occur in those vaccinated. Even so, the U.S. Office of Public Health and Science has recommended that health care workers and others who have the potential for exposure to smallpox be vaccinated.

Other biologic agents

Another possible biologic agent is plague, caused by Yersina pestis (commonly referred to as "Y. pestis"). It can cause either pneumonic plague or bubonic plague, depending on the method of transmission. Bubonic plague can only be spread by the bite of an infected flea or if a person comes in contact with infected material. Pnuemonic plague, a disease of the lungs, concerns health and other officials more, as the bacterium can be aerosolized and then spread from one individual to another by coughing or direct contact.

Y. pestis occurs naturally and could be isolated and grown in the laboratory in large quantities for use as a weapon of mass destruction. The material could be aerosolized and spread across a wide area. Infected persons may not know that they have been infected for as many as six days after the initial exposure.

As a result, they could infect many other people, including individuals in different parts of the country should they travel during that time period.

Also note that antibiotics, when given within seven days of the first signs of infection can be very effective against plague. Left untreated, the bacterium causes illness and death.

The list of other agents used as bioterrorism weapons is long and consists of bacterial agents, such as Cholera, E. coli, and Botulism toxin. Of course, our concerns and imaginations have run wild since September 11, and whether any or all of these agents could be effectively used to infect or kill large numbers of people is unclear.

What is clear is that as a safety director you must retain a level head about the potential for harm and injury that these materials pose. It is true that you will not be working alone should contaminated or infected patients come to your hospital's emergency department. You will be a part of a team working in combination with physicians, epidemiologists, infection control professionals, and nurses. Be an effective part of the team by having the proper knowledge for dealing with these challenges at your immediate disposal.

Besides biologic agents, chemical agents are also under scrutiny. It is in this arena—perhaps even more that the bio-agents—that safety personnel must step up and take a leading role in effectively recognizing the hazard and providing effective methods and tools for protecting employees and patients in the hospital while also dealing with the decontamination of affected patients.

CHAPTER 9

Chemical agents: A long list

As with the biologic agents, the list of chemical agents is long. In addition, chemical agents have unfortunately been used successfully as weapons of mass destruction in the past, while new agents are still being developed and tested. There are several classes of chemical warfare agents, such as neurotoxins, blistering agents, arsines, hydrogen cyanide, and psychotomimetic agents.

Perhaps the best-known chemical warfare agent is the World War I chemical "mustard gas." Mustard gas, named this because of its yellow color and mustard-like smell, is a blistering agent. Exposure does not lead to a high mortality from acute injury. Instead, mustard gas exposure results in long-lasting disability, disfigurement, and pain.

Mustard gas causes severe blistering of the skin, eyes, and mucous membranes. If inhaled, mustard gas causes severe damage to the lungs. Complications of this lung damage can ultimately lead to death. In addition, mustard gas can damage cellular DNA leading to the development of cancer in those who are exposed and birth defects in the offspring of those exposed.

The Treaty of Versailles in 1919 banned Germany from using mustard gas as a chemical weapon. The Geneva protocols banned the use of chemical weapons, and currently 65 nations are shaping a new treaty to ban the use of chemical weapons.

Iraq used mustard gas extensively in the Iran-Iraq war between 1979 and 1988, resulting in the death of an estimated 5,000 Iranian soldiers. Mustard gas is relatively easy and inexpensive to produce, and is therefore a likely first choice for those who wish to develop an arsenal of chemical weapons.

The powerful organophosphates, which have long been known to be neuro-toxins (a chemical that causes harm or injury to nervous tissue), are among the chemical agents developed for use as weapons of mass destruction. Sarin gas and VX are two of those agents. Sarin gas is 26 times more lethal than cyanide gas and 20 times more lethal than potassium cyanide (an adult lethal dose of Sarin gas is equal to 0.01 milligram/kg of body weight).

The Nazis first produced Sarin gas in 1939 for use in the extermination camps. Most recently, a terrorist cult group in Japan in 1995 used Sarin gas. Members of the group timed the release of the gas in three separate subway lines during morning rush hour. About 640 people suffered some effect of the gas, two of whom died.

Sarin gas is colorless, odorless, tasteless, and diffuses very rapidly into the human skin. Sarin affects nerve function by interfering with the mechanism of nerve cell transmission. This type of nerve cell interference can be deadly, leading to loss of such routine functions as breathing.

VX was originally developed as a pesticide. However, it was soon discovered that it was also very toxic to humans. As a result, the U.S. federal government banned its use. VX, like Sarin, is an organophosphorous-based neurotoxic agent. Interestingly, however, no one has yet attempted to use VX as a chemical weapon because of the fact that the gas is so lethal and uncontrollable, that release would cause death not only to the target group, but also to the perpetrators.

As mentioned, other chemical agents have also been developed for use as weapons of mass destruction. Among these are LSD-like chemicals, which can cause psychotic reactions, thus the term "psychotomimetic." These agents have not, to anyone's knowledge, been used as chemical weapons to date. However, they have the potential for use as chemical weapons in small environments with selected targets.

Beware the 'dirty bomb'

Finally, we are all too familiar with the deadly effects of nuclear weapons, such as the atomic bombs used to end World War II. As safety professionals, we also know the effects that exposure to or ingestion of radioactive materials containing strong alpha or beta energy can produce, including cancer, cellular defects, and perhaps heritable genetic defects. It is here that a somewhat new generation of nuclear weapon threatens, namely, the development of a so-called "dirty bomb."

This weapon will not create massive destruction or death. Instead, the generation of psychological fear among the population makes it a potent weapon. The dirty bomb is actually a combination of low-level radioactive materials, such as those containing alpha- and beta-emitting compounds, and an explosive. It has been suggested that used radioactive compounds from medical applications could be included to create a dirty bomb. The concept would be to spread contamination over a relatively narrow area. This could create, more than anything, havoc and fear.

In summary, biological, chemical, and radioactive materials have all either been used or thought of as weapons of mass destruction. In some instances, the mass destruction is really localized—even focused—harm or injury that could, as with Anthrax, result in death.

Each of these elements could spur a great deal of fear and anxiety among the public. They also lead to a need for hospitals and the safety staff to be prepared to deal with those who may come to the hospital contaminated or believing that they have been contaminated with a dangerous agent. You need to know how to deal with the issues of contamination to prevent the potential spread of the agent and further contamination of the hospital environment.

Decontamination procedures

Become familiar with the best methods for protecting staff and other employees who come in direct contact with contaminated or potentially contaminated patients.

Emergency response personnel have been trained to decontaminate on the scene before allowing exposed victims to enter an ambulance. Although they are usually very conscious of this requirement, it is possible for exposed victims to slip through or for victims to transport themselves to the hospital. In that instance, emergency personnel should alert hospital staff ahead of time that an exposed victim is likely on his or her way to the hospital.

Train staff to prevent exposed victims from just walking in to the emergency room, including directing them to a designated decontamination area. This not only applies to bioterrorist attacks, but any incident in which hazardous materials could cling to the clothing, skin, hair, etc., of an exposed person. Asbestos exposure is a classic example of such a situation.

In addition, since the first point of contact for exposed victims in these situations could be security or even a receptionist at the front entrance, include them in your training.

Unless you can verify that exposed victims were decontaminated at the scene, decontamination must take place before they enter your facility. This poses a number of potentially daunting logistical challenges.

In order to make the planning and training a success, nurses and physicians need to participate in the pre-planning and practice sessions. They can help you in answering questions that you cannot answer without their help. For example, other types of injuries could occur at the same time as the chemical, biological, or radiological exposures resulting from an explosion. Consider the following questions:

- Which procedures will be followed to triage the most injured patients even before exposed victims have been decontaminated?

- Who will be assigned to perform the triage (e.g., on-duty emergency room nurse)?

- Should you assemble a designated team specially trained for this type of emergency?

- How will these patients be decontaminated and by whom?

- Are there procedures in place to protect patient privacy and confidentiality (the Health Insurance Portability and Accountability Act of 1996 also applies to patients treated in the emergency room during triage as other parts of the hospital)?

- How will you dispose of contaminated equipment, clothing, and water runoff?

Include hospital staff and ambulance personnel in the decontamination plan. You will probably not get a lot of argument from emergency response personnel who come in on an ambulance, but you might need to convince doctors and nurses who triage exposed patients that they will also need to be decontaminated. Seek support from senior emergency room personnel, including the head physician and nurse, in getting staff to comply with decontamination procedures.

Bioterror and personal protective equipment

Provide training on the use of personal protective equipment. The most difficult aspect of preparing and training staff to deal with contaminated patients is actually getting nurses and physicians to understand the importance of— and the need—to wear such equipment, particularly respirators.

Often, these professionals have been reluctant to use respirators because of their perception that this equipment is frightening for patients, which could interfere with the delivery of the best medical care. They also fear that respirators prevent them from communicating adequately with their patients. Yet for years, these professionals have been accustomed to wearing surgical masks.

Doctors and nurses have also mistakenly believed that these surgical masks can be used to protect them against patients' hazardous materials exposures. The use of a respirator that is High Efficiency Particulate Air filtered at 95% efficiency has gone a long way in educating medical personnel and hospital administrators about the need to use other types of protective devices that go beyond the mere surgical mask.

With the arrival of the potential for other kinds of hazards, move the awareness and education level of personal protective equipment to the next level. Teach doctors and nurses how to properly wear and use this equipment and help them understand how much more effective respirators are than surgical masks to keep them safe from exposure.

Where to turn for information

As discussed previously, you need to understand bioterrorism and how to ready your facility against it. The emphasis that is being placed on emergency preparedness today has given rise to the development and funding of a variety of programs that will allow the safety professional to become knowledgeable about these materials and the ways to recognize and handle them.

Some local communities offer educational and training opportunities. For example, the New Jersey Hospital Association has established a resource site that contains Web sites, literature, books, and audiovisuals for health professionals on emergency preparedness, bioterrorism, and disasters.

The CDC, the National Library of Medicine, and the U.S. Army Medical Research Institute for Chemical Defense has slides and handouts available on these topics.

Local emergency response agencies in cooperation with the Department of Homeland Security, Federal Emergency Management Agency, the Environmental Protection Agency, and the U.S. military also provide educational material and hands-on training and drills. The Internet is a rich resource for finding sites dealing with information about weapons of mass destruction and their hazards.

And finally, professional organizations such as the American Industrial Hygiene Association and the American Society of Safety Engineers offer seminars and programs to train their members about terrorism and emergency preparedness.

Chapter 10

OSHA Recommendations for Ergonomics Compliance

Introduction

Ergonomics has been a hot topic for some time now within the health care industry. In 2000, at the very end of Clinton's tenure in office, he signed into law, by way of an executive order, the OSHA Ergonomic Proposed Rule. Shortly after that, when President Bush assumed the White House, the Senate and House repealed the law, viewing it as flawed.

At the same time, Congress enacted legislation that prevented OSHA from trying to redesign or reintroduce legislation that in any way resembled the just repealed law. Not only was the law seen as flawed, it also created many rifts between management and labor on issues surrounding ways to prevent ergonomic or musculoskeletal disorders (MSDs). Also, political parties were unable to resolve how to pay for changes in the workplace. Even so, the newly elected leadership recognized the need to create some form of federal guidance, if not legislation, to deal with these types of injuries.

The ergonomics problem was an interesting one. Many industries, even without federal intervention, had been showing significant reductions in the number of reported ergonomic-related injuries during the previous 10 years. One glaring exception was the health care industry, particularly the nursing home segment. In fact, ergonomic injuries were the leading cause of injuries and lost work time in nursing homes, according to the Bureau of Labor Statistics. Acute care hospitals were not far behind.

New Secretary of Labor Elaine Chao, and the new head of OSHA, John Henshaw, met with stakeholders and conducted public meetings around the nation before devising a unique strategy to tackle to ergonomics problems. Their tactic involved a four-pronged approach to ergonomics, explained shortly, that would help employers and employees resolve the problem of MSDs, which include cumulative trauma disorders, repetitive motion disorders, and other work-related injuries due to ergonomics.

You need to be at the forefront of efforts to develop an effective ergonomics program. Examine the injury and illness rates and lost work time statistics for your facility. You will discover that, just like in the nursing home, a hospital's highest incident and lost work time rates are in the area of ergonomic injuries. In addition, it will not be surprising to learn that the highest percentage of injuries occurs among the largest segment of the work population in your facility: nurses. Even so, there are other groups who are also susceptible to ergonomic injuries, such as housekeepers and maintenance personnel.

Ergonomics involves such disciplines as anatomy, physiology, psychology, occupational hygiene, and industrial engineering. The discipline of ergonomics is the attempt to fit workplace conditions and job demands with the capabilities of the working population. When performed correctly, workers are more productive at their jobs. At the same time, employees reduce the chances of injury and illness because ergonomics lessens their exposure to job hazards.

There are a number of work-related injuries that can be classified as ergonomic or MSDs These include low back pain, sciatica, rotator cuff injuries, epicondylitis, and carpal tunnel syndrome. These injuries can result from repetitive movement, incorrect lifting or reaching, twisting while lifting, or working at a computer in an incorrect, and often uncomfortable, position.

Every workplace is different. The OSHA guidelines for prevention of these injuries can be applied or modified as the work conditions dictate to improve the quality of employees' work environment and reduce MSDs.

Historical perspective: The four-pronged approach

At the outset, OSHA's four-pronged approach to ergonomics included the following:

- The development of guidelines
- An enforcement policy
- OSHA outreach and assistance
- Research

Nursing homes and long-term care facilities were singled out as prime targets for the development and application of the first set of ergonomic guidelines. Nursing homes were targeted not only because of the high incidence of ergonomic injuries, but also because it was believed that there were effective controls available to resolve many of the sources of these injuries. Thus, focusing on the ergonomic hazards would help reduce the high rate of injuries and illnesses in this segment of the health care community.

Note that many of the problems and challenges the nursing home industry faces are also found in the acute care setting. Similarly, the means of resolving these hazards are also available to the acute care hospital.

The following is the four-pronged approach to ergonomics in detail, as announced in 2002:

Guidelines

OSHA will lead the initiative to develop industry- or task-specific guidelines that are based on current incidence rates and available data about effective and feasible solutions for ergonomic problems. The development of guidelines will, in part at least, take into consideration guidelines and best practices that other industries have already developed. The meat packing industry, for example, established a set of ergonomics guidelines in 1990. These guidelines were effective in reducing MSDs in that industry and, as OSHA officials were happy to point out, without the development of regulatory requirements.

At the time OSHA announced the four-pronged approach, it was also the agency's intention to develop and release the guidelines as rapidly as possible. Part of the reason for this was to demonstrate that this approach could be quickly and effectively put into place, while also directing efforts to reduce workplace injuries in nursing homes and long-term care facilities due to ergonomic hazards.

Enforcement

OSHA indicated that it would concentrate its enforcement efforts in the area of ergonomics on problem employers who continued to experience a high rate of ergonomic injuries. Specifically, OSHA would target employers who did not take positive steps to develop an effective ergonomics program and who did not institute changes to protect workers from these injuries. Since there was no regulation that OSHA could use to cite uncooperative employers, it was committed to using the "general duty clause" as a means of enforcement. The clause, which falls under Section 5(a)(1) of the Occupational Safety and Health Administration Act, states that the employer failed to create a work environment free of recognized hazards. Violations of the act can result in penalties ranging from a minimum of $5,000 up to a maximum of $70,000 per violation. OSHA would perform inspections of facilities based on the highest rate of injuries and lost work time related to ergonomics. The facilities that were among the worst performers would receive an ergonomic hazard alert, making them subject to a follow-up inspection within 12 months after the letter was issued.

It is interesting to note that in 2003, OSHA introduced a National Emphasis Program on ergonomic hazards that included acute care hospitals and nursing homes. OSHA issued hospitals ergonomic hazard alert letters, conducted inspections, and conducted subsequent inspections within 12 months.

OSHA's intention, however, was not to be punitive, but to help resolve ergonomic issues. Therefore, OSHA would provide specialized training to its staff on ergonomic hazards and abatement methods. The agency plans to designate 10 regional ergonomic coordinators who will be involved in enforcement and outreach. In this way, those employers with a high percentage of MSDs will receive help from OSHA.

OSHA developed the ergonomics plan as a compilation of guidelines, rather than a set of standards or regulations. The idea was to provide flexibility for employers in developing new and creative ways of complying with methods to reduce ergonomic injuries in their facilities.

Outreach and assistance

As mentioned previously, OSHA intended to provide assistance to the regulated community to help them proactively address ergonomics issues in the workplace. This assistance would be in the form of advice and training on the voluntary guidelines and implementation of an effective ergonomics program. In order to meet this commitment, OSHA had announced several initiatives, beginning with the designation of a portion of its fiscal year 2002 training grant funds to address ergonomics issues. Added to that, OSHA would develop a complete set of compliance assistance tools. These tools include Internet-based training and information to help employers better understand the guidelines in order to develop an effective ergonomics program. Courses would be made available at OSHA's 12 nonprofit educational partner sites, known as the Education Centers, to make training available to a wider audience. The agency would also develop distance-learning programs.

To develop and highlight the value and effectiveness of the ergonomics guidelines, OSHA would develop new partnerships and sites already recognized by the Voluntary Protection Program (VPP), an OSHA outreach program. Volunteers from the VPP sites would be asked to mentor and train others.

OSHA would establish recognition programs for those employers who successfully develop and implement effective ergonomics plans. The program recognizes those employers who set a high standard for health and safety. Public announcements about a company's contribution and success are the typical rewards. To get there, companies must go through a rigorous inspection process and receive a clean bill of health.

Finally, special attention would be paid to help those workers with limited capabilities in English, especially Hispanic and other immigrant workers.

Research
OSHA will act as a catalyst to stimulate research into areas of ergonomics where information gaps exist. OSHA's intention was also to form an advisory committee to identify research gaps related to ergonomics and the application of ergonomics in the workplace. This committee will report its findings to the assistant secretary and to the National Institutes for Occupational Safety and Health (NIOSH). Using this information, research would be conducted to help fill these information gaps and to develop new methods for reducing or eliminating ergonomic hazards. OSHA would seek collaboration in these research efforts between NIOSH and the National Occupational Research Agenda.

Ergonomic guidelines for nursing homes

In March 2003, OSHA released the final version of the guidelines, or as they refer to them, recommendations, to assist members of the nursing home and personal care industry to reduce the number and severity of MSDs. OSHA was quick to point out that these guidelines would be effective not only for nursing homes and long-term care facilities, but also for other similar work environments, more specifically acute hospitals and other types of health care settings.

The guidelines for reducing ergonomic or MSDs turned out to be a compilation of simple, commonsense applications of patient lifting techniques and carrying and transfer techniques. A commitment by management to ensure that there is an effective ergonomics program in place was the finishing touch. A portion of management assistance can come from having functional equipment in place to meet the challenges faced by long-term care providers on a daily basis.

Nursing home occupants, as well as patients in hospital settings, are often reliant on their care provider to assist them with all of their routine daily tasks, including walking, bathing, or even moving up in bed. The injuries that health care providers can develop are the result of the large number of physical demands placed upon them as they do their jobs. Some of the demands that they face include the following:

- The weight of the patients when being moved or lifted
- The awkward postures that result from them leaning over a bed or working in a confined area
- The shifting of weight that may occur if a resident loses balance or strength while moving

The risk factors for MSDs to employees working in health care have been identified as the following:

- **Force**—the amount of physical effort required to perform a task (such as heavy lifting) or to maintain control of equipment or tools
- **Repetition**—performing the same motion or series of motions continually or frequently
- **Awkward postures**—assuming positions that place stress on the body, such as reaching above shoulder height, kneeling, squatting, leaning over a bed, or twisting the torso while lifting

Guidelines for patient lifting and repositioning

OSHA's guidelines for ergonomics state first and foremost that whenever it is feasible, eliminate manual lifting of residents. Failing that, minimize manual lifting to the greatest extent possible by use of proper mechanical aids. In addition, management should institute an effective ergonomics process that includes the following:

- **Management support**—The best way for management to show its support is to develop clear goals, assign responsibilities to designated staff members to achieve those goals, provide necessary resources, and ensure that assigned responsibilities are fulfilled.

- **Employee involvement**—Employee involvement is a key component of the ergonomics process. Employee participation adds problem-solving capabilities and hazard identification assistance, enhances worker motivation and job satisfaction, and leads to greater acceptance when changes are made in the workplace.

There are a variety of ways to stimulate employee participation in the ergonomics program, such as having employees discuss the workplace and work methods; involving employees in the design of work, equipment, procedures, training, and equipment evaluation; having workers respond to employee surveys; allowing them to participate in task groups with responsibility for ergonomics; and getting them involved in the development of the ergonomics program.

• **Problem identification**—Develop systematic methods for identifying ergonomics concerns in the workplace. Use a variety of information sources, such as OSHA injury and illness logs or workers' compensation claims. Analyze and evaluate that data to identify those tasks that are more frequently associated with ergonomic injuries. Since some of this information may contain restricted or sensitive information, be prepared to take a leadership role in collating and analyzing the data. Next put it in a format that can be effectively shared with employees to develop strategies to reduce or eliminate problems encountered in various locations.

As part of the process, include identification of units or work areas with the highest rates of ergonomic injuries. If you lead inspections of these areas, you can highlight the tasks that lead to injuries. Of course, include in these site visits representatives from other departments, such as nursing and occupational health and administration.

• **Implementation of solutions**—Once you identify the problems, lead brainstorming sessions to develop solutions to the problems. These solutions may involve workplace modifications to eliminate the hazards or improvement of working conditions, such as the introduction of the use of mechanical aids and/or new work practices.

When selecting methods for lifting and repositioning residents, take a variety of factors into account. Include factors such as the patient's rehabilitation plan, the need to restore the patient's functional abilities, medical contraindications, emergency situations, and patient dignity and rights.

- **Rapidly addressing reports of injuries**—MSDs need to be handled in the same way that you handle other injury and illness reporting and investigations. Report injuries as soon as possible. Investigate the event with the nurse manager on the unit where the injury occurred as quickly as possible. Diagnose the employee's injury quickly. One of the most common types of interventions in ergonomics injuries is an alternative duty program. This program allows injured employees to remove themselves from the work environment so that they can limit the severity of the injury, improve the effectiveness of treatment, minimize the likelihood of disability or permanent damage, and reduce the amount of associated workers' compensation claims and costs.

- **Training**—Integrate ergonomics training into the facility's general training on performance requirements and job practices. Effective training addresses the specific ergonomic issues found in each type of job to help reduce MSDs. Conduct this type of training in collaboration with the physical therapy and occupational health departments.

- **Continuous improvement**—Evaluation and follow-up of ergonomics problems and their solutions are central to continuous improvement and long-term success. In addition, evaluation helps sustain the effort to reduce injuries and illnesses, track whether ergonomic solutions are working, identify any new problems, and show areas where further improvement is needed. A good way to perform a follow-up evaluation is to interview employees and seek their input once a new technique has been introduced. Other ways of tracking changes is to once again review the facility's OSHA injury and illness logs and workers' compensation claims.

Patient lifting and repositioning tasks can be variable, dynamic, and unpredictable in nature. When considering what techniques are best suited for patient lifting or repositioning, a variety of factors need to be taken into account, such as resident dignity, safety, and medical contraindications. (See Figure 10.1 for an example of an ergonomics policy for patient lifting.)

The resident assessment should include examination of factors such as the following:

- The level of assistance the patient requires
- The size and weight of the patient
- The ability and willingness of the patient to understand and cooperate
- Medical conditions that may influence the choice of methods for lifting or repositioning

A patient needs' evaluation will not only help determine the best methods to use for patient lifting and repositioning, it will also provide employees with the information they need to do the job safely and with less chance of an MSD. A variety of standardized approaches to the patient needs' evaluation have been published (see Figure 10.2). These charts address many of the challenges encountered with patient lifting and repositioning.

The role of the safety officer

As has been pointed out elsewhere in this book, safety is everyone's responsibility. You cannot be everywhere all of the time. However, you can provide the leadership, stimulate the thought processes, and initiate the development of policies and programs that can percolate throughout the organization to help everyone understand the importance of, in this case, ergonomics injury prevention. Employees also need to understand the importance of their active participation in the process of program development.

Education is one of your key responsibilities. As such, lead this effort by putting together a program that will educate employees about the hazards of ergonomics injuries and how to prevent them. Clearly, there are probably others in the hospital who have a great deal of knowledge in the areas of proper body positioning for lifting and patient movement. These people must be brought in to the process to ensure that a team of the most knowledgeable people conducts the training.

Other hospital staff members must also be brought onto the team. Even though you need to be at the helm, the cooperation of other members of the staff is essential to make sure that everyone accepts the program and has the full support of all segments of the hospital population. Some of the key players include the director of nursing, members of senior administration, and the occupational health nurse.

Figure 10.1

Sample Ergonomics Policy for Safe Patient Lifting and Repositioning

(Note: The following policy is from the *Patient Care Ergonomics Resource Guide: Safe Patient Handling and Movement*, Patient Safety Center of Inquiry, Veterans Administration and the Department of Defense, April, 2002.)

Purpose: To describe methods that ensure that safe techniques are used for when assisting patients who need to be moved or repositioned.

Policy: _____ is committed to providing the highest quality of care for its patients. At the same time, _____ is also committed to maintaining a safe and healthful work environment for its employees. To assist in this effort, a Back Injury Prevention Program has been implemented. Appropriate support is available to help employees meet the standards set for safe patient lifting and repositioning. The program also includes the proper equipment necessary for safe patient lifting and repositioning. In order to ensure that the program is successful, employee training, patient care needs assessment and evaluation of the ergonomic risks associated with all tasks on all units are evaluated and analyzed. Manual lifting of patients should be avoided under normal circumstances; mechanical devices should be used to assist employees when lifting or moving patients. The only exception is when a medical emergency precludes the use of such equipment.

Responsibilities:

Administration:
- Support implementation of the lifting policy
- Ensure that mechanical lifting and repositioning devices are available in sufficient numbers and locations
- Make certain that equipment is properly maintained
- Ensure that new equipment is purchased when needed

Figure 10.1

Sample Ergonomics Policy for Safe Patient Lifting and Repositioning (cont.)

Supervisors:

- Support implementation of policy
- Ensure that employees are properly trained in patient care lifting, repositioning, and in the hospital's patient lifting and repositioning policies
- Participate in evaluation of equipment and patient assessments
- Ensure that mechanical lifting devices are available and in good repair
- Promptly report employee injuries to Occupational Health
- Maintain OSHA injury log
- Ensure that injured employees participate in Back Injury Prevention Program

Employees:

- Become familiar with and comply with patient lifting and repositioning policies
- Participate in patient assessments and risk evaluation
- Participate in appropriate training
- Report injuries promptly

Procedures:

Compliance:

Employees responsible for their own health and safety, and must also ensure that patient care and patient safety needs are met. Compliance with all parts of this policy is an important component in achieving these goals.

Safe Patient Lifting and Repositioning:

- Assess and evaluate all patient lifting and repositioning requirements before doing them.

Figure 10.1

Sample Ergonomics Policy for Safe Patient Lifting and Repositioning (cont.)

- Avoid situations in patient lifting and repositioning that may result in injury to the employee or the patient.
- Use mechanical lifting devices and other approved patient handling equipment under normal circumstances. Medical emergencies may constitute an exception.

Training:

Employees are required to participate in health and safety training programs at the time they are hired and periodically thereafter. A portion of the program will include education about the facility's safe patient lifting and repositioning policies and procedures. Training will also include information concerning the proper use of mechanical devices for patient lifting and repositioning. Training will also occur each time new equipment is purchased and brought into the facility.

Back Injury Prevention Program:

A back injury prevention program will be implemented under the auspices of the Occupational Health Department. The program will include the following:
- Ergonomic workplace assessment
- Use of lifting devices and equipment
- Education in patient assessment techniques to ensure proper patient lifting and repositioning
- Methods to prevent back injuries
- Education techniques to use when back rehabilitation is needed
- Follow-up review and evaluation

Incident/Injury Reporting:
- Ergonomic injuries should be promptly reported to supervisors and Occupational Health
- Incident reports should be promptly completed

Figure 10.2

Patient Needs Evaluation Outline

(**Note:** The following evaluation outline is from the *Patient Care Ergonomics Resource Guide: Safe Patient Handling and Movement,* Patient Safety Center of Inquiry, Veterans Administration and the Department of Defense, April 2002.)

Patient Needs Evaluation Outline

In order to effectively manage the ergonomics issues that surround patient lifting and repositioning, a patient needs evaluation should be developed to determine the best methods to use for patient lifting and respositioning. Such a needs evaluation will also provide workers with the information they need to do the job safely and with less chance of an MSD. The following are examples of the relevant issues that must be addressed in a patient lifting and repositioning assessment:

1. Transfer of patients to and from: bed to chair, chair to toilet, or chair to chair.
   a. Considerations include
      i. Can patient bear weight?
      ii. Is the patient cooperative?
      iii. Does the patient have upper extremity strength?

2. Lateral transfer to and from: bed to stretcher
   a. Considerations include
      i. Is caregiver assistance required and to what extent?
      ii. Weight of patient.

3. Transfer to and from: chair to stretcher
   a. Considerations include
      i. How cooperative is patient?
         a. full body sling lift and two caregivers

Figure 10.2

Patient Needs Evaluation Outline (cont.)

           ii. Can the patient bear weight?

               a. Non-powered stand assist may be sufficient

4. Reposition in bed: side to side, up in bed
   a. Considerations include
      i. Can patient assist?
      ii. Weight of patient.
      iii. Use of friction devices, positioning aids.
      iv. Involve several caregivers to avoid injuries.

5. Reposition in chair: wheelchair or dependency chair
   a. Considerations include
      i. Is patient cooperative?
      ii. Can patient assist?
      iii. Does chair recline?
      iv. Can chair move?

6. Movement of patient up from floor
   a. Considerations include
      i. Was patient injured?
      ii. How severe was injury?
      iii. Can patient assist in getting up?

Develop interdisciplinary teams consisting of nurses, nursing supervisors, nurse managers, physical therapists, and physicians to perform patient evaluations. A key member of the team will be the employee(s) directly responsible for patient care and assistance. As the needs and abilities of patients typically vary, even over a short period of time, the employees responsible for providing assistance are in the best position to be aware of and accommodate such changes.

Setting an ergonomics program in motion

The place to begin this process is with the safety committee. As suggested in Chapter 6, use the safety committee as both a sounding board and as a support group for safety programs.

Inform the committee members about the types of initiatives and efforts that can be put in place to help change the numbers and prevent employee injuries. The reduction in lost work days and workers' compensation time will also not be lost on the safety committee nor the administration that must struggle with budgets and the cost of paying workers' compensation claims and lost workday insurance policies.

Once the committee has endorsed the ergonomics injury reduction initiative, put an education program in place. Employees from all sectors of the organization need to hear about the program and what it will mean to them. They also need to know what role they will play in the program's success.

One of the important components of an ergonomics program is the need to eliminate or reduce as much as possible the necessity of lifting patients. There needs to be a commitment on the part of administration and employees to develop cooperative lifting teams. In addition, administration must commit to putting money into the purchase of adequate lifting devices and mechanical aids. The safety committee can be very helpful in accomplishing both of these tasks.

Resources

As mentioned previously, there are a number of OSHA resources, including educational programs and Internet training sites. Also, within the typical hospital, there are many different individuals, including physical therapists and occupational health nurses, who have experience with patient movement techniques and injury prevention programs.

In addition, there are now many organizations, such as the American Association of Occupational Health Nurses that have launched a Web site, *www.ergoresources.org*, designed to aid occupational and environmental health professionals access a number of free, online ergonomics resources. In addition, the U.S. Veteran's Administration publishes information dealing with ergonomics issues.

Perhaps the most important resources to use in developing an ergonomics program for your facility are those available within your facility, such as your injury and illness logs and the past year's workers' compensation claims. Use the expertise in your hospital to evaluate and analyze the sources of these injuries and to develop strategies to reduce or eliminate them. The frontline employees are probably the most valuable resources available to you as you conduct a needs evaluation and survey your facility to find the units and work areas that need the attention first.

OSHA mechanical device recommendations

OSHA recommends the following use of various types of mechanical devices when lifting and repositioning patients:

1. Transfer from sitting to standing position

Powered sit-to-stand or standing assist devices are recommended for use when transferring patients who are partially dependent, have some weight-bearing capacity, are cooperative, can sit up on the edge of the bed with or without assistance, and are able to bend hips, knees, and ankles. This type of transfer involves movement of patients from bed to chair (wheelchair, Geri or cardiac chair), or chair to bed, or for bathing and toileting. These devices can also be used for repositioning where space or storage is limited.

Such devices come with a variety of sling sizes, a wide range of lift-height capabilities, battery portability, hand-held controls, an emergency shut-off, and manual override. Make sure the device is rated for the resident weight. Electric/battery powered lifts are preferred to crank or pump type devices to allow smoother movement for the patient, and less physical exertion by the caregiver.

2. Patient lifting

A portable lift device (sling type) or a universal/hammock sling or a band/leg sling is a possible solution to the problem of lifting patients who are totally dependent, are partial- or non-weight bearing, are very heavy, or have other physical limitations. These devices can be used for transfers from bed to chair (wheel chair, Geri or cardiac chair), chair or floor to bed, for bathing and toileting, or after a patient fall.

More than one caregiver may be needed to safely use such a device. When buying these devices, look for those that come with a variety of slings, lift-height ranges, battery portability, hand-held control, emergency shut-off, manual override, a boom-pressure sensitive switch that can easily move around equipment, and a support base that goes under beds. Having multiple slings allows one of the slings to remain in place while the patient is in bed or in a chair for only a short period, thus reducing the number of times the caregiver lifts and positions the patient. Portable compact lifts may be useful where space or storage is limited. Ensure that the device is rated for the resident weight. Electric/battery powered lifts are preferred to crank or pump type devices.

Another tool that can be used for patient lifting is a ceiling mounted lift device. As with the portable lift device, this can be used to lift patients who are totally dependent, are partial or non-weight bearing, very heavy, or have other physical limitations. A horizontal frame system or litter attached to the ceiling-mounted device can be used when transferring residents who cannot be transferred safely between two horizontal surfaces, such as a bed to a stretcher or gurney while lying on their back, using other devices.

More than one caregiver may be needed to safely use this device. However, some patients may be able to use the device without assistance. The ceiling mounted equipment may be quicker to use than the portable device. Motors can be fixed or portable (lightweight). This lifting tool can be operated by a hand-held control attached to the unit or by infrared remote control. Ensure that the device is rated for the patient weight.

3. Walking

An ambulation assist device is designed for use by patients who are weight bearing and cooperative and who need extra security and assistance when walking.

The ambulation assist device increases patient safety during movement and reduces risk of falls. The device supports residents as they walk and push it along during movement. It is critical to ensure that the height adjustment is correct for the patient before walking is allowed. Also, the caregiver must ensure the device is in good working order before use and that it is rated for the patient weight to be lifted. Remember to apply the brakes before positioning a patient in or releasing a patient from the device.

4. Lateral transfer/Repositioning

A possible solution to the problem of repositioning a patient in bed or transferring a partial or non-weight-bearing patient between two horizontal surfaces, such as from bed to stretcher, is the use of a draw sheet or transfer cot with handles in combination with slippery sheets, low-friction mattress covers, or slide boards. Boards or mats with vinyl coverings and rollers, gurneys with transfer devices, and air-assist lateral sliding aid or flexible mattress inflated by a portable air supply can also serve the same purpose.

As in other situations, more than one health care worker is needed to perform this type of transfer or repositioning. Additional assistance may be needed depending upon patient status, e.g., for heavier or noncooperative residents. However, some devices may not be suitable for the extremely heavy patients

(>250 pounds). When using a draw sheet combination use a good handhold by rolling up draw sheets or use other friction-reducing devices with handles such as slippery sheets. Narrower slippery sheets with webbing handles positioned on the long edge of the sheet may be easier to use than wider sheets. When using boards or mats with vinyl coverings and rollers use a gentle push and pull motion to move the resident to the new surface.

In order to increase patient comfort and minimize the risk of skin trauma, try to find a combination of devices that will serve the function. Make sure that transfer surfaces are at the same level and at a height that allows health care providers to work at waist level to avoid extended reaches and bending of the back. Count down and synchronize the transfer motion between caregivers.

5. Repositioning in chair

Use a variable-position Geri or cardiac chair when repositioning partial- or non-weight-bearing patients who are cooperative.

Typically, more than one health care provider is needed and use of a friction-reducing device is needed if the patient is unable to assist in repositioning him- or herself in the chair. Be sure that caregivers use good body mechanics while performing the task. The work will be facilitated when there are wheels on the chair, the chair is easy to adjust, move, and steer. For safety purposes, lock the wheels on the chair before repositioning and remove trays, footrests, and seat belts where appropriate. Be sure that the chair is rated for the patient weight.

6. Lateral transfer in sitting position

Transfer boards, some with movable seats, are suggested for transferring patients who have good sitting balance and are cooperative from one level surface to another, such as bed to wheelchair, wheelchair to car seat or toilet. Patients who require limited assistance but who need additional safety and support can also use these devices.

Movable seats increase patient comfort and reduce the incidence of tissue damage during transfer. More than one health care provider is needed to perform a lateral transfer. Reduce trauma to the skin by making sure that there is clothing present between the patient's skin and the transfer device. The seat may be cushioned with a small towel for comfort. This type of device may be uncomfortable for larger patients. Such devices are usually used along with gait belts for safety depending on patient status. Make sure boards have tapered ends, rounded edges, and appropriate weight capacity. Make sure wheels on the bed or chair are locked and transfer surfaces are at same level. Remove lower bedrails from the bed and remove arms and footrests from chairs, as appropriate.

7. Transfer from sitting to standing position

Lift cushions and lift chairs are recommended for transferring patients who are weight-bearing and cooperative but who need help when standing and walking or when an independent patient needs an extra "boost" to stand.

Lift cushions use a lever that activates a spring action to assist residents to rise up. Lift cushions may not be appropriate for heavier patients. Lift chairs are operated by a hand-held control that tilts forward slowly, raising the patients. Patients need to have physical and mental capacity to be able to operate lever or controls. Always make sure that the device is in good working order before use and that it is rated for the weight of the patient who is to be lifted. These devices can help aid patient independence.

An alternative to the lift cushion or lift chair is a stand-assist device that can be attached to the bed or a chair. The stand-assist device can also be freestanding. The device must be stable before use and must be rated for the weight of the patient who is to be supported.

8. Weighing

There are a number of devices that can be used to weigh non-weight-bearing or totally dependent patients. Scales with a ramp to accommodate wheelchairs, a portable powered lift device with built-in scales or a bed with built-in scales will help reduce the need for additional lifting and transfer of patients. Some wheelchair scales can accommodate larger wheelchairs. In some cases, built-in bed scales may increase the weight of the bed and prevent it from lowering to appropriate work heights.

9. Transfer from sitting to standing position and walking

Gait belts or transfer belts with handles can be used when transferring patients who are partially dependent, have some weight-bearing capacity, and are cooperative, from bed to chair, chair to chair, or chair to car. Such tools may also be effective when repositioning patients in chairs, supporting patients during ambulation, and, in some cases, when guiding and controlling falls or assisting a patient after a fall.

When using gait belts or transfer belts with handles, more than one health care worker is often needed. Belts with padded handles are easier to grip and increase security and control. Always transfer to patient's strongest side. Use good body mechanics and a rocking and pulling motion rather than lifting when using a belt. Belts may not be suitable when helping heavy patients to walk or move or in cases of patients who have had recent abdominal or back surgery, abdominal aneurysm, etc. Belts should never be used for lifting patients.

When using the belt, make sure it is securely fastened and cannot be easily undone by the patient during the transfer. Make sure there is a layer of clothing between the patient's skin and the belt to protect the skin from injury. Keep the patient as close as possible to the health care provider during the transfer. Lower bedrails; remove arms and footrests from chairs, and other items that may obstruct the transfer.

After a fall, always assess the patient for injury prior to moving him or her. If the patient can regain a standing position with minimal assistance, use gait or transfer belts with handles to aid resident. The health care provider who is performing the lift should always keep his or her back straight while bend the legs, and staying as close to the patient as possible. If the patient cannot stand with minimal assistance, use a powered portable or ceiling-mounted lift device to move the patient.

10. Repositioning

An electric powered, height-adjustable bed is recommended for use in all activities involving patient care, transfer, repositioning in bed, etc., in order to reduce the amount of bending that the health care provider must perform.

These devices should have easy-to-use controls that are located within easy reach of the health care provider to ensure the use of the electric adjustment, sufficient foot clearance, and a wide range of adjustment. Adjustments must be able to be completed in 20 seconds or less, as this helps make sure that the staff will use them.

For patients who may be at risk of falling from the bed, beds that lower closer to the floor may be needed. Heavy-duty beds are available for excessively overweight patients. Beds raised and lowered with an electric motor are preferred over crank-adjust beds to allow a smoother movement for the patient and less physical exertion by the health care worker.

Patients with upper body strength who are able to readily use their extremities and who are cooperative and can follow instructions, should be allowed to use trapeze bars, hand blocks, and push-up bars attached to the bed frame for movement and repositioning.

Patients who are able can use trapeze bars suspended from an overhead frame to raise themselves up and reposition themselves in a bed. Heavy-duty trapeze frames are available for excessively heavy patients. If a health care worker is helping the patient, make sure that bed wheels are locked, bedrails are lowered, and that the bed is adjusted to the worker's waist height.

Blocks also enable patients to raise themselves up and reposition themselves in bed. Bars attached to the bed frame can serve the same purpose, although this may not be suitable for heavier patients.

Pelvic lift devices (hip lifters) can be used to assist patients who are cooperative and can sit up to a position on a special bedpan. The use of this type of device may reduce the need for patient lifting during toileting. The device is positioned under the pelvis. The part of the device located under the pelvis is inflated, thus raising the pelvis and allowing for a special bedpan to be placed underneath. The head of the bed is raised slightly during this procedure. To ensure safety, the health care provider needs to use correct body mechanics, lower bedrails, and adjust the bed to his or her waist height to reduce bending.

11. Bathtub, shower, and toileting activities

Use a height-adjustable or easy-entry bathtub when bathing patients who are able to sit directly in the bathtub. This equipment can also be used to assist ambulatory patients to climb more easily into the tub. Patients can be placed in a tub for bathing using a portable-powered or ceiling-mounted lift device outfitted with an appropriate bathing sling.

Using these types of aids reduces awkward postures for health care workers, as well as for those who clean the tub after use. The tub can be raised to eliminate bending and reaching. Using correct body mechanics, and adjusting the tub to the worker's waist height when performing hygiene activities can significantly reduce injuries to the worker. These aids can also increase patient safety and comfort.

Height-adjustable shower gurneys or lift bath carts with waterproof tops are available for use when bathing non-weight-bearing patients who are unable to sit up. The patient should be transferred to a cart with lift or lateral transfer boards or other friction-reducing equipment. The cart can then be raised to eliminate bending and reaching for the health care worker. Foot and head supports are available for patient comfort. This technique may not be suitable for excessively heavy patients. Make sure the carts that are purchased are power-driven to reduce the amount of force that will be needed to move and position the device.

Built-in or fixed bath lifts are recommended for bathing patients who are partially weight bearing, have good sitting balance, have upper body strength, are cooperative, and can follow instructions. These aids are also useful in small bathrooms where space is limited.

When using these tools, be sure that the seat rises so the patient's feet clear the tub, easily rotates, and lowers the patient into the water. Again, this tool may not be suitable for heavy patients. Always check to make sure that the lifting device is in good working order before use and that it is rated for the proper patient weight. Choose a device with a lift mechanism that does not require excessive effort by the health care worker when raising and lowering it.

Shower and toileting chairs are for use with patients who are partially dependent, have some weight-bearing capacity, can sit up unaided, and are able to bend hips, knees, and ankles. Before using the chairs make sure that the wheels move easily and smoothly and that the chair is high enough to fit over the toilet, has removable arms, adjustable footrests, safety belts and is heavy enough to be stable.

Also, the seat should be comfortable, able to accommodate larger patients, and have a removable commode bucket for toileting. Also check to make sure that the brakes lock and hold effectively and that weight capacity is sufficient. Bath boards and transfer benches are the equipment of choice for bathing patients who are partially weight bearing, have good sitting balance, can use their upper extremities, are cooperative, and can follow instructions. Independent patients can also use these devices.

When using these aids, use clothing or material between the patient's skin and the board to reduce or eliminate injuries to patient skin. These devices can be used with a gait or transfer belt and/or grab bars to aid transfer. Back support and vinyl-padded seats add to bathing comfort. The optimal devices will allow for water drainage and will have height-adjustable legs. These devices may not be suitable for heavy residents. If a wheelchair is used, ensure that the wheels are locked, the transfer surfaces are at the same level, and that the device is securely in place and rated for the weight to be transferred. Remove arms and footrests from chairs, as appropriate, and ensure that the floor is dry.

Toilet seat risers are for toileting partially-weight-bearing patients, who can sit up unaided; have upper body strength; are able to bend hips, knees, and ankles; and are cooperative. Independent patients can also use these devices. When using these aids, risers decrease the distance and amount of effort required to lower and raise patients. Grab bars and height-adjustable legs add safety and versatility to the device. Ensure that the device is stable and can accommodate the patient's weight and size.

Grab bars and stand assists that may be fixed or mobile are among the other types of mechanical aids that can be effective in toileting or bathing patients. Long-handled or extended showerheads, or brushes can be useful for personal hygiene. Such equipment helps reduce the amount of bending, reaching, and twisting that the health care worker must do when washing a patient's feet, legs, and trunk. Independent patients who have difficulty reaching lower extremities can also use these devices.

In addition, movable grab bars on toilets minimize workplace congestion. Be sure that bars are securely fastened to the wall before use. Bars and assists help when toileting, bathing, and/or showering patients who need extra support and security. Remember, patients must be partially weight bearing, have upper body strength, and be cooperative.

Ergonomic hazards found in other health care jobs

There are other types of work activities that take place in hospitals beyond patient lifting and repositioning. Some of these tasks include cleaning floors, collecting trash, restocking supplies, serving and delivering meals, and handling laundry chores. These jobs may also be a significant source of MSDs. Similar to the process described for patient care providers, a job hazard analysis needs to be performed for each of these tasks. Again, employee involvement and management commitment are required to reduce or eliminate the ergonomic hazards associated with these jobs.

Some of the problem areas and recommended solutions include the following:

1. Storage and transfer of food, supplies, and medications

- Use carts when moving food trays, cleaning supplies, equipment, maintenance tools, and dispensing medications
- When placing items on the cart, keep the most frequently used and heavy items within easy reach between hip and shoulder height
- Carts should have full-bearing wheels of a material designed for the floor surface in your facility
- Carts should have wheel locks
- Carts should have handles that are vertical, with some horizontal adjustability that will allow all employees to push at elbow height and shoulder width
- Handles should be able to swing out of the way, which can save space or reduce reach.
- Heavy carts should have brakes
- Loads should be balanced and under cart weight restrictions
- Ensure stack height does not block vision
- Low profile medication carts with easy-open side drawers are recommended to accommodate hand height of shorter nurses

2. Mobile medical equipment

Use mobile carts, wheeled devices to transport equipment, for example:

- Oxygen tanks: use small cylinders with handles to reduce weight and allow for easier gripping. Secure oxygen tanks to transport device.
- Medication pumps: use stands on wheels.
- Equipment: push, rather than pull equipment

Keep arms close to the body and push with whole body and not just arms. Remove unnecessary objects to minimize weight. Avoid obstacles that could cause abrupt stops. Place equipment on a rolling device, if possible. Place defective equipment out of service. Perform routine maintenance on all equipment.

When moving and transporting patients, make sure additional equipment such as oxygen tanks and IV/medication poles are attached to wheelchairs or gurneys or moved by another caregiver to avoid pushing awkwardly with one hand and holding freestanding equipment with the other hand.

3. Working with liquids

Housekeeping

Use buckets on wheeled devices for easier moving without the need to lift or carry the bucket. Make sure the bucket has a faucet for easy emptying. These devices are most useful in housekeeping areas when filling and emptying buckets with floor drain capabilities. This type of set-up reduces risk of spills, slips, speeds process, and reduces waste. Be sure that wheels don't get stuck in floor grate. Use a hose to fill the bucket. Be sure to maintain the wheels in good condition.

Kitchens

When filling and emptying liquids, such as soups or other liquid foods, into or from containers use an elevated faucet or hose to fill large pots and a ladle to empty pots. Small saucepans can also be used to dip liquids from pots. Avoid lifting heavy pots filled with liquids. If the worker stands for more than two hours per day, shock-absorbing floors or insoles will minimize back and leg strain. With hot liquids, use a splashguard.

4. Hand tools

Make sure to select and use properly designed tools that fit the grip and are properly sized and weighted for the job and the user. Make sure a regular maintenance program is in place. Use bent-handled tools, when appropriate, to avoid wrist bending, and choose tools that have minimal vibration or built-in vibration reduction devices. Always make sure proper personal protective equipment is used.

5. Linen carts

Use spring loaded carts that automatically bring linen within easy reach when moving or storing linen. Be sure that the spring tension of the cart is appropriate for the weight of the load. Carts should have wheel locks and height-appropriate handles that can swing out of the way. Heavy carts should have brakes.

6. Handling bags

When handling laundry, trash and other bags, use receptacles on wheels that have side openings that keep the bags within easy reach and allow the employees to slide the bag off of the cart without lifting. Chutes and dumpsters should be positioned to reduce or minimize lifting. Remember, it is better to lower the chute or dumpster than to lift the materials to a higher level. Minimize awkward handling and testing by providing automatic opening or hardware to keep doors open.

7. Reaching into sink

Tools can be used to modify a deep sink when it is being used to clean small objects. Such tools include a plastic basin in the bottom of the sink to raise the work surface. An alternative is to use a smaller porous container to hold small objects for soaking, transfer to an adjacent countertop for aggressive cleaning, and then transfer back to the sink for final rinsing. Store inserts and containers in a convenient location to encourage consistent use. This technique is not suitable in kitchens/food preparation.

8. Loading or unloading laundry

The use of front-loading washers and dryers speeds the process for retrieving and placing items, and minimizes wear-and-tear on linen. Washers with tumbling cycles separate clothes, making removal easier. For deep tubs, a rake with long or extendable handle can be used to pull linen closer to the door opening. Raise machines so that the opening is between hip and elbow height of employees.

If using top-loading washers, work practices that reduce risk include handling small loads of laundry, handling only a few items at a time, and bracing your body against the front of the machine when lifting. If items are knotted in the machine, brace with one hand while using the other to gently pull the items free. Ensure that items go into a cart rather than picking up baskets of soiled linen or wet laundry.

9. Cleaning rooms

Wet method

The following are recommendations when cleaning rooms with water and chemical products; and using spray bottles:

Cleaning implements use: alternate leading hand; avoid tight static grip and use padded nonslip handles.

Spray bottles: use trigger handles long enough for the index and middle fingers. Avoid using the ring and little fingers.

For all cleaning

- Use chemical cleaners and abrasive sponges to minimize scrubbing force.
- Use kneepads when kneeling

- Avoid bending and twisting
- Use extension handles, step stools, or ladders for overhead needs
- Use carts to transport supplies or carry only small quantities and weights of supplies
- Ventilation of rooms may be necessary when chemicals are used
- Avoid lifting heavy buckets, e.g., lifting a large, full bucket from a sink
- Use a hose or similar device to fill buckets with water
- Use wheels on buckets that roll easily and have functional brakes
- Ensure that casters are maintained
- Use rubber-soled shoes in wet areas to prevent slipping

10. Cleaning wheelchairs: Cleaning workstation should be at appropriate height.

11. Electrical methods

The recommended work methods and tools for vacuuming and buffing floors are as follows:

- Both vacuum cleaners and buffers should have lightweight construction, adjustable handles, triggers (buffers) long enough to accommodate at least the index and middle fingers, and easy to reach controls.

- Technique is important for both devices, including use of appropriate grips, avoiding tight grips and for vacuuming, by alternating grip. The use of telescoping and extension handles, hoses and tools can reduce reaching for low areas, high areas and far away areas. Maintain and service the equipment and change vacuum bags when 1/2 to 3/4 full.

• Vacuums and other powered devices are preferred over manual equipment for moderate-to-long duration use. Heavy canisters or other large, heavy equipment should have brakes.

Finally, as in most situations, training is a key component of the ergonomics programming. Provide training to all workers in a language and method that is readily understandable. Also, offer training to those who will be responsible for the development and implementation of the ergonomics program, as well as the workers who must perform the tasks.

The guidelines recommend the following training components:

Train employees before they lift or reposition patients, or perform other work that may involve risk of injury. Include ergonomics training with other safety and health training. Training should include case studies or demonstrations based on the hospital's policies, and should allow enough time to answer employee questions.

At a minimum, training should ensure that workers understand the following:

• Policies and procedures that should be followed to avoid injury, including proper work practices and use of equipment

• How to recognize MSDs and their early indications

• The advantages of addressing early indications of MSDs before serious injury has developed

• The hospital's procedures for reporting work-related injuries and illnesses as required by OSHA's injury and illness recording and reporting regulation (29 CFR 1904).

Charge nurses and supervisors should reinforce the facility's safety program, oversee reporting guidelines, and help ensure the implementation of patient- and task-specific ergonomics recommendations, e.g., using a mechanical lift.

Because nurses and supervisors are likely to receive injury reports, and are usually responsible for implementing the hospital's work practices, they may need more detailed training than nursing assistants. Such training should include

• methods for insuring use of proper work practices

• ways to respond to injury reports

• ways to help workers implement solutions

Staff members who are responsible for planning and managing ergonomics efforts need training so they can identify ergonomics concerns and select appropriate solutions. These staff members should receive information and training that will allow them to do the following:

- Identify potential problems related to physical activities in the workplace through observation, use of checklists, injury data analysis, or other analytical tools
- Address problems by selecting proper equipment and work practices
- Help other workers implement solutions
- Evaluate the effectiveness of ergonomics efforts.

Chapter 11

Laboratory Safety

Hospital laboratories, whether their mission is clinical or research, pose a number of challenging issues for you. A large part of your work and responsibility today involve issues of laboratory safety. The first step is to understand the differences between clinical and research laboratories.

Research laboratories, on the other hand, try out a variety of often-untested new procedures using a number of different chemicals. Although researchers try to reach a point in their research where procedures for a series or set of protocols can be standardized for each new experimental trial, this level of standardization is often not achievable. Arriving at the end point of a series of experiments often involves a circuitous path of previously untested and untried procedures.

Clinical laboratories, on the other hand, use methods and techniques that have been clearly defined and spelled out by various clinical oversight groups, such as the American Society of Clinical Pathologists. These methods usually have no variations or testing required on the part of the laboratory once these groups accept them and enter them into the practice standards. While the clinical laboratory worker may use hazardous materials or hazardous procedures, these materials and methods have been standardized to such an extent that the hazards have been either very clearly defined or, at the very least, minimized.

Research laboratory workers perform experiments at all hours of the day and night, often with little or no oversight or supervision by the researcher or by senior laboratory personnel. Clinical tests may also be performed at any time, depending on the size of your facility and the nature of the services your hospital provides. However, the technical staff usually closely monitor these tests.

Thus, both types of laboratory environments, clinical and research, raise a variety of concerns for the safety director, including the following:

- Safe use of chemicals
- Establishing and maintaining a database of hazardous materials and material safety data sheets (29 CFR 1910.1200)
- Complying with OSHA's Laboratory Standard (29 CFR 1910.1400)
- Electrical safety
- Hazardous waste storage and disposal
- Training

Clinical labs are often easier to deal with from the safety director's perspective because of the routine nature of the work, the degree of control over the work, and the standardization of the procedures (fewer untested methods are used). As an example, the use of chemicals is more standardized and routine in the clinical laboratory as compared to the research laboratory. This situation allows the laboratory personnel to more readily manage chemical usage through chemical tracking and development of a solid base of material safety data sheets, which is often more limited in number than in the research laboratory.

Also, chemical waste storage and disposal is more straightforward and, under existing EPA regulations, easier to handle in clinical laboratories than in research laboratories. The EPA allows for the establishment of a satellite waste site in the laboratory, with the collection of up to 55 gal of any particular waste stream. Since clinical laboratories use fewer and more defined waste streams, this requirement is more easily met in clinical laboratories than in research laboratories. This situation is true even in clinical laboratories that use a variety of chemicals, such as the anatomic pathology laboratory, even though the volume of chemicals in each waste stream is much larger than in the chemistry lab.

Finally, in many clinical laboratories, such as chemistry or immunology, the use of premixed kits reduces the volume of waste chemicals generated and lessens the chance of spills or incorrect mixing of materials. In addition, the high-tech equipment in use in today's clinical laboratories calls for very low volumes of both reagents and test materials in order to perform tests that give accurate results. The volumes are often measured in microliters.

Chemical use and storage issues

As stated previously, research laboratories will be more challenging for you. Researchers at these facilities, depending on the nature of the work, can use a wide array of chemicals over a very short period of time as the needs of the experiments become better developed. Often, a particular chemical may be purchased and used only once. Researchers are notorious in their desire to save money, which, in and of itself, is not a bad thing. However, this can lead to bigger expenses and even larger safety problems if the remaining chemical, no matter how low the probability that it will ever be used again, is kept "just in case."

Keeping the remaining chemical on-site may create a problem and lead to the development of a serious hazard. There are some chemicals, for example, that once opened and exposed to light and air, can form explosive peroxides. Isopropyl alcohol, for example, only three months after it is first opened has the potential to become an explosive and therefore is dangerous if the next user is unaware that the material has been opened and left on a shelf.

Such chemicals must be disposed of prior to the three-month expiration date. If not, removal of the chemical can lead to a hazardous removal procedure, including detonation and disposal. Such a procedure can also result in great expense to the laboratory for the costs associated with removal, detonation, and disposal. Accompanying these costs will be the hidden expense of lost research time, as local authorities may need to close down the laboratory until the removal occurs. Even keeping chemicals that do not turn into explosive materials can pose a risk and a large expense to the institution at the time of disposal.

Often, an evaluation is needed to help researchers understand that purchasing smaller volumes of chemicals, even at a higher cost, is cheaper in the long run than purchasing large volumes of chemicals with a greater disposal price tag.

The point of this discussion is to provide you with some ideas and insights on how to better manage the challenges you face in the laboratory, whether research or clinical. Although not everyone may agree about all of the merits of OSHA's involvement in laboratory safety, it does provide help in organization and tracking of hazardous chemicals via two of the OSHA standards: Hazard Communication Standard (29 CFR 1910.1200) and the Occupational Exposure to Hazardous Chemicals in Laboratories, 29 CFR 1910.1450, known as the "laboratory standard." The former regulation requires, among other things, that a material safety data sheet accompany all hazardous chemicals used in the laboratory.

When an appropriate tracking and notification system is devised, the Hazard Communication Standard can assist you in getting a handle on the volumes, locations, and types of hazardous chemicals, including flammables, poisons, corrosives, etc., found in your facility. The laboratory standard states, once again, that material safety data sheets need to be maintained to identify all hazardous chemicals in the laboratory. It also reaffirms the need to train all laboratory personnel in laboratory hazards.

However, the standard also states, among many other requirements, that a chemical hygiene plan is essential for each laboratory, and that each laboratory needs to appoint personnel who are responsible for the administration of the plan, including a chemical hygiene officer and, in some cases, a chemical hygiene committee. The chemical hygiene plan, which needs to be reviewed annually, should describe the methods for safe use and handling of hazardous materials in the laboratory. The plan should also contain standard operating procedures for the use, handling, and disposal of hazardous chemicals.

Other components of the chemical hygiene plan should include the approval of the laboratory director, laboratory manager, and supervisor for the plan; a description of ways that chemical exposures will be monitored; and the means and frequency with which laboratory equipment, such as fume hoods and biosafety cabinets, will be tested and certified to ensure optimal performance. Fume hoods should be tested at least annually, and biosafety cabinets may be tested annually, or more frequently depending on the nature of the materials being used and processed in the cabinet.

Establish a safety presence in the laboratory

Use the requirements of the laboratory standard to establish a clear safety presence in the laboratory, whether clinical or research. Take the lead in helping the laboratories in understanding the requirements of the laboratory standard and the requirements of the chemical hygiene plan. Communicated with the chiefs of service and/or the directors of your facility's various laboratories.

Conduct face-to-face discussions with them to get their buy in and approval of the chemical hygiene plan. Make sure that they accept the responsibility for safety in their laboratories. But let them know that you and the safety staff are there to help and guide them. This can be a delicate process since some laboratory directors and supervisors are not inclined to have "outsiders" intrude in their laboratory operation in any way. This method of gaining support works well because you do not want to interfere with their laboratory operations or procedures. Instead, you just want to be informed and knowledgeable about their workings and understand which hazardous chemicals they use in the laboratory on a regular basis.

Depending upon the circumstances, a chemical hygiene officer and chemical hygiene committee may be appointed for each laboratory or for the entire facility. Once your facility fills those posts, make contact with the officer or chair of the committee to introduce yourself and your staff. In a large organization with several laboratories, this may be a very large undertaking. Nevertheless, let them know that you are there to help them prepare a chemical hygiene plan.

You may also ask to be appointed as a member of the chemical hygiene committee so that you will be a part of the team, and those responsible for the laboratory plan will be a part of your team. Membership on the chemical hygiene committee will also give you, or a member of your staff, an opportunity to review the chemical hygiene plan and the hazardous materials used in the laboratory on a routine basis.

If you work in a smaller facility, you may be appointed the chemical hygiene officer. In that case, laboratory representatives should be selected to assist you by serving on the chemical hygiene committee. Appointments should be made in collaboration with the chief of service or the laboratory director and the laboratory supervisor. Often those who are selected for the committee initially feel that the work is an added burden to what is already a busy workday. But if handled correctly, these appointees can be made to feel that they are part of a productive team that is helping their laboratory and coworkers to stay ahead of problems and safety challenges. Periodic review of the members of the chemical hygiene committee also helps members feel that they are not trapped, and, if they desire, there is a way out.

Another recommendation based on the chemical hygiene officer model is to have the chief of service or laboratory director appoint a laboratory safety officer. This individual can be someone different from the chemical hygiene officer. This person will then function as the primary contact between you, or a representative of your staff, and the individual laboratories. The laboratory safety officer should also be expected to communicate to others in the laboratory and the head of the laboratory about ongoing safety issues and safety concerns, not only in the individual laboratory, but also within the hospital itself. For example, if the fire department has a concern about safety training and will be making inspections of the hospital, you can establish a quick call or e-mail list to notify the safety officers about what is happening.

The appointment of laboratory safety officers and chemical hygiene officers as safety links can be used effectively in both clinical and research laboratories. Clinical laboratories may wish to consolidate all of their safety officers into one committee or group, headed by the laboratory supervisor or chemical hygiene officer. You can then be a member of that committee and provide information and guidance. As distinct from the clinical laboratories, the research laboratories in your facility will probably want to have their safety officers or chemical hygiene officers act independently.

Regardless of the model devised, hold monthly meetings with the laboratory safety officers to discuss problems and issues that arise in the laboratories. The research laboratory officers can all meet together with you as one group, and the clinical personnel as another separate group. In either case, these safety officers can provide you with valuable input and feedback about policies and procedures that are in effect or that you are planning to put into place. Also, use the laboratory safety officer meetings to establish training goals and training criteria and to make sure that all laboratory personnel understand these goals and criteria.

The laboratory safety officers can also help you effectively carry out routine inspections of the laboratories and provide follow-up and resolution of problems in the laboratory. This is why department head and laboratory director approval are so important, since these tasks cannot be resolved without their ultimate support.

Once issues are resolved, request feedback from the safety officers within a reasonable time frame. They can assist in setting up a schedule of laboratory visits and establishing the list of items that you might be looking for during these inspections. This type of collaboration can go a long way in creating a strong safety presence and a viable safety culture in an organization. Of course, the success of the program depends, in part, at least, on your ability to communicate effectively and honestly with the laboratory personnel and their safety officers.

Be willing to listen, take advice, and even a little criticism, from time to time. Although there are a variety of regulatory requirements from local, state, and federal agencies, there may be more than one way to achieve the goals of laboratory safety and worker protection. Do not compromise your principles, but be willing to listen alternative ways to achieve the goals that you and your hospital are trying to reach.

Finally, there are some other indicators that can help you understand what is happening in the laboratories that may cause safety problems, including a material safety data sheet. It should be your responsibility to view the material safety data sheet as it comes into the facility. Know where the listed chemicals are going and who will be using them. Make sure that the laboratory staff members involved in the use of those chemicals have been properly educated about the safe use, handling, and disposal of those materials.

This aspect of your job should not wait until the annual surveillance rounds in the laboratory or until the chemical hygiene plan is reviewed. Make this an ongoing review. Another way to become knowledgeable of the chemicals being used in your hospital is to carefully track hazardous chemical waste disposal. Do the types and volumes of chemicals going out of the laboratory match those that are coming in? Knowing this can help you to better understand the needs of the laboratories. It will also indicate what may be an important expense area for the hospital: chemical waste disposal.
Using surveillance lists for laboratories is helpful in keeping those areas safe. Figure 11.1 is an example of a checklist that can be modified to meet your requirements.

Figure 11.1

Sample Laboratory Surveillance Checklist

Fume hoods have all been checked and certified within the past 12 months.   Y__ N__

Biosafety cabinets have been checked and certified according to department
policy (at least within the past 12 months).   Y__ N__

Material safety data sheets are maintained and up to date.   Y__ N__

The chemical hygiene plan is prepared and reviewed at least annually.   Y__ N__

Laboratory areas that use carcinogens have been properly labeled.   Y__ N__

Personnel training records are up to date.   Y__ N__

Chemical waste satellite disposal areas are clearly marked.   Y__ N__

Waste collection containers are marked with starting date and
waste stream.   Y__ N__

Fire extinguishers are in place and have been properly checked   Y__ N__

The laboratory has conducted fire drills.   Y__ N__

Aisles are clear and free of obstruction.   Y__ N__

Doorways and means of egress are not blocked.   Y__ N__

Figure 11.1

Sample Laboratory Surveillance Checklist, (cont.)

Eye wash and deluge showers are accessible and checked for proper operation.	Y__ N__
Extension cords are not in use.	Y__ N__
Laboratory personnel are using the correct personal protective equipment	
including Lab coats	Y__ N__
Gloves	Y__ N__
Protective eyewear	Y__ N__
Face shields	Y__ N__
Warning labels for hazardous materials, including biohazards, are properly placed.	Y__ N__
Emergency phone numbers are readily accessible.	Y__ N__
Flammable materials are properly stored in safety cabinets.	Y__ N__
Volumes of liquid flammables do not exceed limits allowed by hospital or fire department guidelines.	Y__ N__

Chapter 12

Construction Safety and Project Oversight

One of your most challenging tasks is overseeing a construction or renovation project. Renovation projects are routine events, and can involve everything from rewiring the nursing station for new telephone or computer lines to remodeling patient rooms to upgrade the plumbing or lighting.

The good news about these types of renovations is that the hospital's own maintenance employees typically perform the work. They generally know the hospital, the locations involved, and the prime people to contact about the project. Similarly, the floor staff members usually know which men and women are performing the renovation.

This familiarity helps make your job a bit easier during what can often prove to be trying times. There are precautions that need to be taken and assurances that need to be made to prevent any type of untoward event that could adversely affect patients or employees during renovation. For example, if the nursing station is being renovated to add wiring for the new telemetry system, dust could be raised, asbestos may be discovered above the ceiling tiles and need removing, and the job could be noisy. Even though the workers are hospital employees, they are, nevertheless, "outsiders" who are making their presence felt on the unit for several days. All of these factors contribute to the potential for chaos and disharmony, not to mention hazards for patients and employees alike, during the course of the project.

Construction safety 101

When larger renovation and construction projects, such as remodeling an entire wing of a hospital, renovating and upgrading the operating suite, or taking down an existing building adjacent to a working part of the hospital and replacing it occur, then the disruption to hospital routine and to patients and staff is clearly greater. The construction crew may have never worked in a medical setting before and may have no knowledge of any of the hospital routines or concerns. It also probably doesn't know who any of the important players are on the unit or around the hospital in general.

These workers often do not have a clear idea of the hazards that they might create as they demolish old structures, rip down aged ceilings, or uncover aging water pipes behind closed walls. They may have years of experience with the materials they work with but no knowledge of the hazards they create for others, particularly debilitated patients.

For example, these workers typically have an understanding of the hazards of asbestos, but they probably do not have a full grasp of health care staff and other hospital employees' concern when they remove asbestos or perform work near asbestos that could release fibers into the air. Nor do these workers likely have a clear grasp of the disruption they create just by being there, or by creating noises or vibrations at awkward times, such as during clinical rounds or x-ray examinations.

They certainly do not understand the effects that the equipment and materials they use may have on hospital employees and patients. Often these workers are uninformed about the hazards and disruption they can cause by uncontrolled release of welding fumes, chemical odors from paints and glues, and the release of odors from old pipes carrying waste or even water supplying fire sprinklers. And although information about the release of mold from above ceilings has been discussed at some length over the past several years, construction crews may still be unaware of the role they play in releasing that mold in the hospital. Frequently they consider such complaints by hospital staff a nuisance with no real basis. They probably do not comprehend the serious consequences that such dust and mold release can have on immunocompromised patients or staff members with allergies.

When problems crop up during a construction or renovation project, as almost certainly they will, you typically will receive the call. But there are steps you can take to reduce the frequency of calls and also ease the concerns of hospital staff. At the same time, you can help prevent patient and employee exposures to dust and debris and nuisance odors and harmful materials.

Establishing a preconstruction risk assessment

The JCAHO clearly spells out some of the first steps in that process. Over the past couple of years, the JCAHO has come to the realization that preconstruction risk assessments are an essential element in helping to prevent or reduce the incidences of patient and employee exposure to dust and mold. These requirements actually grew out of recommendations from the AIA and the CDC that highlighted the importance of such assessments. Both organizations recommend that hospital officials form a preconstruction risk assessment. This team should be composed of a range of people from different disciplines such as safety, nursing, administration, infection control, maintenance, the construction manager, and housekeeping to name a few.

The prime requirement, now enforced by the JCAHO, is that this team be assembled prior to the start of any construction or renovation process. The team should identify all of the susceptible patient populations in the hospital and those that might be affected directly or indirectly by the project. This preconstruction risk assessment team should also identify areas in the hospital that house the most susceptible patients, such as operating rooms, transplant units, and cardiac intensive care units, to name a few. The JCAHO thrust was for patient safety, particularly when patients may be exposed to infectious disease hazards such as mold.

The team, although created at the start of the project, should continue to meet regularly throughout the project and even after the completion of the project until such time as a final report and analysis of the team's efforts can be completed and delivered to senior administration. It is also important to note that from an oversight perspective, Joint Commission surveyors will be checking for evidence of the existence of a preconstruction risk assessment team and for verification that it has been meeting and making recommendations. (See Figure 12.1 for an example of a construction safety risk assessment team checklist.)

Figure 12.1

Construction Safety Risk Assessment Team Checklist

Has a preconstruction risk assessment team been selected?   Y__ N__

Members of the team, departments, phone numbers:

_____

_____

Meeting Schedule _____

Hospital Project Manager: Name _____   Phone number _____
Pager _____

Names of hazardous materials and products to be used, along with their material safety data
sheets, have been provided to the risk assessment team.   Y__ N__

Educational information about hospital policies and procedures, emergency plans,
and fire safety plans have been prepared for nonhospital workers.   Y__ N__

Plans for unexpected service interruptions have been prepared and reviewed.   Y__ N__

Floor representatives have been briefed on the construction/renovation project. Y__ N__

Routine meetings with hospital project manager are scheduled.   Y__ N__

Meeting agendas and reports attached
(highlight areas of concern requiring more in depth review).   Y__ N__

Although it is not stated in the JCAHO guidelines, or in the AIA or CDC recommendations, this preconstruction risk assessment should go beyond a concern for mold exposure and infectious disease examination. The efforts of this team should be part of a larger hospital environmental risk analysis. The team would not only review infection control issues, but would also evaluate items such as services that might be interrupted during the project, including water and electricity. For example, team members might help to plan or devise back-up procedures in the event of an unscheduled interruption of services due to a pipe rupture or steam line break. The team members would review for safety the equipment being used and the materials, including paints and chemicals.

Your role in this area is clear. Among other things, review the hazardous components of the chemicals and whether the chemicals can be used safely in the facility, evaluate storage issues for solvents and flammables, and assess plans for setting up containment areas and negative pressure isolation rooms. You are part of the team.

Your other responsibilities

Ensure that the employees from the maintenance department or from an outside contractor have been properly trained and are up to date on their training in such matters as respirator use. Outside contractors should not be allowed to work in the facility until they have received appropriate training from their employer or their union, whoever is most appropriate to provide it, and can demonstrate such proficiency to your satisfaction.

You must make sure that the contractor's employees are properly trained in the hospital's emergency plans, such as fire safety and emergency evacuation. In addition, you, along with the infection control professional, should educate both hospital employees and outside contractors on the procedures necessary to prevent the spread of dust, mold, and construction debris from the work site. These are all considered hazardous for patients and hospital employees.

Work with the hospital project manager and the construction foreman to ensure that proper containment areas and negative pressure isolation areas are set up to prevent spread of dust and debris. Other recommended containment procedures include use of walk-off mats outside of the containment area, disposal of debris in tightly covered dumpsters, and the removal of construction debris only after regular hours and through designated exit routes. In addition, decide ahead of time how to monitor for release of dust or mold, the frequency of monitoring, and responses to an unacceptable release of such materials.

A hospital environmental risk assessment, as an ongoing part of the construction project, should address both patient and employee safety concerns about exposure to molds, chemicals and other types of potential hazards. Inform the health care staff about the project, its goals, expected duration, and the anticipated issues. Provide them with contact information for the hospital project manager, you, or other key personnel who can quickly and effectively address problems.

Asbestos removal is always an issue in older facilities. Before the project begins, conduct an educational forum with affected employees about the asbestos removal project and the steps that will be taken to protect them from any exposures. Such a proactive approach will go a long way to calm fears and reduce calls both to the safety department and regulators. Be involved in selection of companies that perform specialized tasks involving the handling of hazardous materials, such as asbestos.

You need not and should not be alone in overseeing the construction project. Early in the project, hospital officials should appoint a project manager for the oversight of the day-to-day operations on the construction site. If hospital maintenance personnel are performing the project, the department head or a supervisor may be obvious choices.

Work as a team

When an outside contractor is going to be doing the work, then it is just as important, if not more important, that a hospital representative, often the head of maintenance, but sometimes other personnel who have been specifi- cally hired to perform such oversight tasks, are appointed. These individuals should be a part of the preconstruction risk assessment team. They should also help the nurses and staff on the unit establish contact and develop a line of direct, usually daily, communication with the personnel performing the ren- ovations and construction.

It is at this level that such issues as timing of events (e.g., water shutdowns, electrical interruptions, and noisy work) can best be discussed and planned. Of course, this process probably will still have a few bumps along the road. However, the ability of both the nurses and the construction foreman to have a name, face, and telephone number or pager number to reach during times of emergency—real or perceived—goes a long way to calm the nerves and ease the tensions that accompany any construction process, especially one in a health care facility.

Selection of a project manager from the hospital will help you. It gives you a person to contact when a problem occurs on the construction site. It also gives the safety department an extra set of hands to train the construction crew about hospital policies and procedures. The project manager can work with the safety director to educate construction personnel about the special safety precautions they need to take to protect both patients and employees from exposure to chemicals and mold. There is now a person to help ensure that construction employees have been properly trained on how to use respirators and other personal protective equipment before they are allowed to enter the job site.

The project manager can help guide the safety department staff through the various aspects of the construction project to make sure that plans are being followed as they were laid out during the preconstruction phase. Of course, if the plans are altered, the project manager can assist the safety personnel in understanding why the changes were made and how the agreed upon precautions have been adjusted.

As safety director, it is important to recognize that the construction or renovation project will proceed at a pace that is beyond your control. The best that you can achieve is an ongoing relationship with the project manager, the construction manager, and the leaders of the unit affected. The use of these resources, along with the other members of the preconstruction risk assessment team, will help you gain perspective and a sense of control over the hazards associated with the construction or renovation project.

Remember to check daily work practices to ensure that Interim Life Safety Measures have been instituted (if required) and to make certain that the work area is locked each night and that hazardous materials, such as flammables, have been properly stored. (See Figure 12.2 for an example of a construction project checklist.)

Figure 12.2

Construction Project Checklist

Workers are properly trained	
Use of personal protective equipment	Y___ N___
Hospital emergency and fire safety procedures	Y___ N___
Hazards associated with release of dusts, fumes, chemicals	Y___ N___
Containment procedures and requirements	Y___ N___
Work area is clearly marked.	Y___ N___
Storage areas are provided for hazardous materials and flammables.	Y___ N___
Work area is cleaned at least daily.	Y___ N___

Figure 12.2

Construction Project Checklist (cont.)

Hazardous materials are locked up each night.   Y___ N___

Interim Life Safety Measures are used when needed.   Y___ N___

Interim Life Safety Measures are communicated to staff when
instituted or when changes are made.   Y___ N___

Monitoring of work area for release of dust or mold is conducted.   Y___ N___

Procedures are in place if a release is detected.   Y___ N___

There is an emergency contact list posted at nurses' station for project
manager/safety director.   Y___ N___

A procedure has been set up to discuss the schedule for noisy
work or work that will create vibrations.   Y___ N___

All nonhospital workers have been given hospital identification badges.   Y___ N___

ID badges are readily visible when workers move through the hospital.   Y___ N___

Material safety data sheets for materials used on the construction work are
on-site and readily available.   Y___ N___

Chapter 13

Keeping Pace With Emerging Safety Issues

IAQ has become a high-profile problem over the past several years, especially in health care institutions. The root of the problem stems from construction done in the early 1970s to shore up energy leaks in buildings by adding extra layers of insulation that, we ultimately learned, tended to trap odors and fumes. Such insulation also prevented the transfer of air in and out of buildings (except through mechanical means), as sealed, inoperable windows in most hospitals have also replaced open windows.

Indoor air concerns in hospitals have also been raised as a result of hazardous chemicals, such as formaldehyde or ethylene oxide, that are used but may not have been properly exhausted. And of course, until quite recently, cigarette smoking, a problem not unique to health care facilities, was also allowed on virtually every floor of the hospital, and even in patient rooms.

Today, we recognize many of these problems, and have devised solutions for them. We have virtually outlawed smoking, devised better exhaust methods for ethylene oxide and formaldehyde releases, and improved the mechanical ventilation systems in hospitals. Yet, IAQ problems remain a concern.

Recently, the CDC released a report[1] that discussed environmental infection control issues in health care facilities. Among the topics of this report was the concern over the spread of mold and infectious agents as a result of certain activities, such as construction.

This is an important concern in health care institutions that house sick and immunocompromised patients who are readily susceptible to many of these organisms, including Aspergillus fumigatus. Some patients, such as transplant patients, could die as a result of such an exposure. Of course, efforts are made to protect patients from these exposures, including the use of HEPA filters on the air supplies to these patient care areas. Operating rooms also have their air supplied through these filters in conjunction with a high air exchange rate in order to help keep the room air clean and free of contaminants.

The variety of IAQ problems

Patients are not the only ones affected by mold and air contaminants. Hospital workers are also subject to the effects of these air intruders. Studies have shown that the rate of asthma in the population at large has increased over the last 20 years, and nurses are not excluded from that increase. Thus, the effects of poor IAQ affect not only patients, but also those who provide those patients with care. Mold, paint odors, cleaning product odors, and chemical smells heighten everyone's sense of awareness and caution. Often times, workers need to be sent home or placed on long-term observation with accompanying medication to overcome the effects of these IAQ problems.

---

[1]. *Guidelines for Environmental Infection Control in Health-Care Facilities*
Recommendations of CDC and the Healthcare Infection Control Practices Advisory Committee
(HICPAC) Prepared by Lynne Sehulster, PhD and Raymond Y.W. Chinn, MD, June 2003

Sometimes the IAQ complaints do not come about as a result of odors or mold. Other times the complaints are due to "bad air" that smells musty or stale. Yet, other times, the criticism comes about because the air is too hot, and occasionally, too cool. Typically, these problems result from ineffective heating ventilation and air conditioning (HVAC) systems. The air circulation may be inadequate, filters may be out of alignment, or, in certain HVAC systems, the drip pans may not have been properly cleaned to remove the buildup of moisture and ultimately, mold. In some cases, the odors emanate from refrigerators or ice machines that have not been properly cleaned and maintained.

Over the past decade, some IAQ complaints have stemmed from another type of allergen: latex. Latex gloves commonly used by surgeons, nurses, and other health care providers contain natural rubber latex. This latex attaches to the powder inside of the glove that helps you put them on and take them off more easily. As the glove is removed, the powder carries the latex particulates with it and employees become affected.

Nurses have a rate of latex allergy that is around 9% nationwide, the highest of any occupational group. Latex allergies can be debilitating under some conditions. To combat this, the concentrations of latex in gloves have been reduced, and in many institutions use of latex gloves has been eliminated entirely. Also, gloves that do contain latex have either switched to containing very low levels of powder or none at all. This has helped reduce the occurrence of latex allergies. Those who are already latex allergic may continue to have problems, however, even when low-latex, powder-free gloves are used. Some hospitals have also established latex-free zones for those employees who are affected by latex.

Tips for handling IAQ problems

IAQ problems, as seen from the previous discussion, encompass a wide array of triggering events. As safety director, you will get the calls and the complaints, and you will need to investigate each of these complaints.

Do not dismiss any complaint. Each one is real in the eyes of the complainant, and what may seem frivolous or unfounded to you is genuine and might have a basis in fact.

At times, the complaints may increase, such as in the fall and winter when the heating system is turned on for the first time that year. Typically, this is the result of the release of odors from the heating system. This can be particularly true if your facility uses steam for heating that contains anticorrosives, such as aminopholines. These chemicals, if contained inside of the steam pipes, go unnoticed; but if there is a leak, as in a radiator valve, many people will notice the odor, and some will actually become ill from the odor.

Make sure that the maintenance department is your close ally in responding to and investigating IAQ complaints, especially as they relate to the HVAC systems.

As mentioned previously, odors from cleaning activities, particularly floor stripping and waxing, are often at the source of indoor air complaints. Many products claim to have reduced or eliminated the chemical components that affects personnel. A regular review of the cleaning products that are used in your facility is a good idea. There are many products that have now been identified as "green products," environmentally safe and free of harmful chemicals to help reduce some of the IAQ complaints.

Align your IAQ activities with your housekeeping department. Work with them to develop a list of approved products for general and floor cleaning use. If there is an individual who has a known history of problems when floor stripping and waxing occurs, plan the work on the night that employee is not on duty, or have the employee assigned to another unit during the expected cleaning time. There are usually only one or two employees in any given area who are highly susceptible to these odors.

Dealing with IAQ issues require a consistent response and an honest effort in order to build staff confidence that you will investigate each event fairly and objectively. You also need to have the proper resources to help you investigate and resolve such complaints.

Form an IAQ committee. Include on the committee department heads or senior members from safety, infection control, maintenance, housekeeping, occupational health, engineering, and human resources. Representatives from other departments, such as nursing, can also be beneficial to the group. The committee should report to the appropriate senior administrator who has the power to provide funds and the resources necessary to resolve any large or hospital-wide IAQ problems, such as the latex allergy issue described previously.

The committee should appoint a chair from safety, occupational health, or any of the other member departments. The committee should meet regularly, keep notes, and be actively involved in investigating and resolving IAQ issues. It is important to keep in the loop the personnel who made the complaint, to provide feedback on the progress and findings, and to seek their input on the matter.

Learn from past

IAQ is not a new issue. Each day, however, new concerns come forward from a variety of sources that you need to be aware of. A few years ago, for example, medical waste incinerators and the disposal of contaminated and infectious waste became a problem. Not only were there concerns about disposal of needles infected by bloodborne pathogens, such as HIV or hepatitis B, there were also fears about the byproducts put into the air and water from the medical waste incinerators that hospitals used to burn this waste. The release of dioxins from the incinerator stacks, and the discharge of mercury from the water effluents used in the incinerator stream, placed a high level of scrutiny on the use of these incinerators and the levels of pollution they created.

The concern over incinerators was finally resolved in most places because the Environmental Protection Agency issued tight restrictions and inspection requirements on the incinerator discharges. The end result was that virtually all the hospital incinerators around the country closed down because the cost of upgrading and maintaining the incinerators in order to keep them compliant with state and federal regulations was prohibitively expensive. At the same time, the cost of medical waste disposal leveled off, making the use of private vendors for medical waste disposal more palatable.

The circumstances surrounding the investigations and studies into medical waste incinerators took several years. You role went from worrying merely about safety inside the hospital to being concerned about the impact that your hospital's operations had on that environment. As a result of the incinerator investigations, another issue came to the forefront. This issue is still on the front burner of hospital safety professionals, administrators, and environmental officials: the use of mercury and mercury-containing products.

Eliminating mercury as a hazard

Mercury is found in a variety of chemicals and products used in the hospital, and is not just limited to thermometers or sphygmomanometers. Dental amalgams and chemicals used in the laboratory, bleaches, soaps, and cleaning products have all been found to contain trace levels or more of mercury.

When disposed of down the drain, this mercury can eventually be absorbed by plants and animals and passed along the food chain to humans. Efforts are underway to eliminate mercury-containing products such as thermometers and sphygmomanometers in hospitals. Hospitals all over the country have conducted high-profile events designed to replace mercury-containing devices with those that contain no mercury. Hospitals have also made efforts to uncover what chemicals contain low levels of mercury so that they can be replaced. In most instances, the safety director is the prime mover in understanding the places where mercury can be found and in helping to determine how to eliminate mercury, or, if that is not possible for technical or other reasons, for preventing the release of mercury into the environment and into the waste stream.

The examples discussed in this chapter highlight the need for the safety director to stay current in a wide range of areas. The two topics mentioned previously both come from the environmental arena. But other areas require your attention, as well. For example, the evolution of an ergonomics process for health care facilities quickly comes to mind. You must participate in ongoing education. Read current literature on the topics and attend meetings and seminars to ensure that you keep pace with the varied number of new developments in the broad area that we call health care safety.

Chapter 14

Education and Training

Introduction

The safety program may be only as good as its education and training component. How can employees work safely and take the necessary steps to comply with safety requirements if they are not both educated and trained about safety?

Employees need to be educated about the hazards associated with various tasks and the reasons that jobs are performed in certain ways. Employees also need to be trained—that is, shown—how to actually perform certain jobs properly so that they avoid injuring themselves or harming others.

Whether it is proper lifting techniques to protect against injury from repeat stress trauma or learning how to properly wear a respirator to protect themselves from exposure to airborne diseases such as TB, workers need to be carefully shown the way to maintain safety. They also need to understand why they take the measures that they do. Employees need to both practice the ways that jobs are done safely and understand why the recommendations are made in a specific manner.

Safety education

Safety education begins for all employees on their first day of work. This education should start with an overview of the entire safety program across the whole hospital. It should describe what employees need to know to work at that hospital and to be a part of the organization. New employees should at this time also understand what their role in the hospital's safety program is and what is expected of them. New employees should see clearly how seriously you and the hospital administration view the safety program and every employee's compliance with that program.

During orientation, there is usually not enough time to give new employees all the information that they need to know to work at their job. Often, safety information gets lost among forms that deal with salary, insurance, and benefits. Therefore, at orientation only the basic outline of the safety program should be given, with instructions about how and when to sit in on the additional training that is required.

Conduct additional training within the first seven to 10 days of employment. Managers and supervisors should ensure that their newest employees receive this training. Additional sessions will most probably include fire safety and fire extinguisher use, a review and explanation of the hazard communication program, respirator fit testing and training for medically cleared employees for TB respirators, and information about workplace violence prevention.

Employees also need individualized education about the specialized tasks they might perform. For example, laboratory personnel will need additional training about safe chemical use and handling, and people who work in material management will need additional instructions about safe lifting techniques to avoid back injury.

In addition, some employees will need education about the special requirements of the location where they work. For example, those who work in the maternity ward or in the psychology unit will have to be educated about the special safety requirements of their location in the event of a fire or, in the case of the maternity ward, in the event of abduction. All employees need to learn about the safety requirements of their work area, such as the location of the fire exits, the fire extinguishers, and any emergency call buttons.

In addition, there should be a way of tracking employees' participation in safety education. Joint Commission surveyors will often look for training records and try to link participation in employee education with a particular employee. The human resources department may be the appropriate place to keep those training records. Training records may also be maintained on the unit where the employee works. However, track employee participation in orientation and in the ongoing education that they receive in safety.

Once orientation takes place and an employee sits through the first series of safety sessions, the training is not over. Safety training should be repeated annually, and there should be a way of linking performance reviews and annual salary reviews to attendance at and participation in safety programs. The responsibility for ensuring that an employee takes part in safety education every year lies with the employee and his or her supervisor. Your role is to make sure that the education is readily available.

You need to provide training to all employees on all shifts. There are, of course, many ways to reach that goal. One of the methods that is becoming more popular, and more effective, is the use of Web-based training programs that employees can participate in when they have the time in their schedule.

A caution is needed here, however. If this type of training is being offered, a great deal of work needs to be done by the safety director to ensure that the safety training is appropriate to the facility. In other words, pre-written programs are usually not adequate, as they do not address the idiosyncrasies of your facility. It would also be appropriate to make sure that someone is available to answer questions that employees have about what they have learned.

Identifying the key elements

To a large degree, the components of safety education in health care are no different from those elements found in other industries. But because of the different role that hospitals have in society, as compared to other businesses, there are added requirements for safety training that must address the issues of maintaining personal safety due to exposure to patients.

Of course, any safety education program must take into account the specific needs of the hospital and its workers. If your facility has confined spaces, then of course this needs to be included in your education program. If you have underground storage tanks (UST) for fuel oil, then education programs dealing with USTs are needed for the employees who work with those tanks.

Other programs are virtually universal in all facilities, such as fire safety, hazard communication, and emergency preparedness. Then, as mentioned, there are the unique programs that hospital employees need: protection against blood-borne pathogens or TB, what to do in the event of an infant abduction, and knowledge about biohazards, radiation hazards, and lasers, to name but a few.

Some elements of safety education are easy to identify because they are mandated by various regulations put forth by OSHA or the EPA. There are other safety education elements, however, that are not necessarily required by any agency but should be included in your safety program. How do you identify these?

These are the programs that come about as a result of your ICES network, or as a result of incident reports that you review, or from surveillance rounds. This is when you learn that OSHA or the Joint Commission requirements really are only basic elements of a safety program. It is a time when you learn that there are many tasks that people need to be educated about in order to prevent injury or harm to themselves or others.

A nonexhaustive list of education and training programs that you might need to consider for your facility might look something like Figure 14.1.

Figure 14.1

Education Programs

- Fire safety
- Laser safety
- Hazard communication
- Hazards of waste anesthetic gases
- Needlestick prevention
- Spill control procedures
- Workplace violence
- Emergency preparedness
- Americans with Disabilities Act training
- Biosafety
- Hazardous materials handling
- Bloodborne pathogens
- Asbestos training
- TB training
- Radiation safety
- Respiratory protection
- Ergonomics hazard training
- Incident reporting techniques
- Electrical safety
- Bomb threat response
- Response to infant abduction

How do you know whether safety education has been effective?

Providing safety education is only half the job. The other half is to make sure that people understand what they have been taught and then put that into practice. But how do you measure this?

Of course, one way is to test people after the course has been completed. Fire safety quizzes are not uncommon (see Figure 14.2 for an example). Other ways of measuring success are less objective, but also effective. One involves a combination of two different techniques: observe employees performing their jobs before and after they have been trained, and review incident reports (this will reflect the types of problems that may be found throughout the hospital).

Often an investigation will show where safety education and training has failed or where employees are merely refusing to follow the safety guidelines that have been given to them. The goal of collecting this information or making a thorough record of observations is not to chastise a particular individual, it is to determine whether the education employees received has gotten through and whether those techniques have been adapted and put into practice.

Figure 14.2

Safety Quiz

Safety tests or quizzes following the training are not uncommon. When designing these tests, the idea is to ask questions to see if people have heard what they have been taught. A safety quiz might look like this:

1. Does the XYZ Hospital have a special code word for fire? What is it?

2. How are fires announced to the hospital?

3. What is your role in fire safety?

4. What kind of fire extinguisher would you use for:
   a. trash fire
   b. electrical fire
   c. chemical fire

5. When do you evacuate a patient?

6. How do you know whether it is safe to come back after a fire?

7. Where is the nearest fire extinguisher to your workstation?

8. Where is the nearest fire exit?

9. What is the telephone number to call in case of emergency?

10. Does the hospital have emergency lights?

Chapter 15

Safety Director Ethics

Consider how to approach your job and determine your place in the hospital environment. You must meet the needs of the hospital, its administration, and governing body to ensure that the facility maintains a high standard of safety and regulatory compliance. In addition, you must meet the needs of the employees and staff to make sure that they are educated and informed about the ways to perform their jobs in the safest way possible with the least risk to themselves and their coworkers.

Performing those duties alone would most likely meet the minimum requirements of the job of safety director, and would probably put you in a good light with respect to hospital administrators and bosses. But there is more to your position than just making administrators and bosses happy.

Professional guidelines

Safety directors come from a number of professional backgrounds, as you might expect. And, no matter what the background, you can almost be assured that there is a professional organization to which a safety director may belong. That organization will most probably have its own guidelines for what it considers to be the best practice behaviors for professional conduct.

The backgrounds and professions that may lead to your position include safety professionals and industrial hygienists, many of whom belong to the American Society of Safety Engineers or the American Industrial Hygiene Association, or both. Both of these organizations publishes guidelines on ethical behavior. Both organizations publish guidelines with statements such as "practice the profession using recognized scientific principles," "maintain up-to-date competency in your area of expertise," "do not try to perform work outside of your area of expertise," "maintain confidentiality," and "perform your work with honesty and impartiality."

These ethical guidelines may seem obvious, yet in today's business world it's easy to lose sight of these targets, which go beyond the mere legal requirements of regulatory compliance or the dictates of your written job description. Although you are employed by an entity, and have a boss to whom you must report, you have a bigger obligation to maintain a high level of integrity to yourself and your own principles and those of ethical professional conduct.

Your first and perhaps most important professional obligation in the work that you perform is to look at each situation objectively and evaluate it based on the facts alone. As an example, consider IAQ complaints that have become a large and not uncommon issue. Often, however, there are those who attempt to stigmatize those employees who complain by belittling them. This is sometimes the case when the people who complain are the nurses who essentially live and work on the unit and are the ones most affected by the air quality problems. Yet, some employees may not view them as credible or consider their complaints valid, particularly the female nurses. Why? Well, some of the reasons that have been given include, "they are more susceptible [to indoor air quality problems]," "they are more delicate," "it is hormones," and finally, a total brush-off: "it is their imagination."

As a safety professional, guided by a set of ethical rules, you need to approach every situation with an independent attitude and an open mind. Collect the data, perform the sampling and testing that is required, and then use that information to determine the truth. It may be difficult, as IAQ concerns can become high profile, rancorous issues, and you may have forces on both sides of the issue pushing you to agree with their perception of the problem.

Some of the players in these situations will often include the complainants, perhaps their union and other interested or sympathetic parties, administrators, and bosses. It can be very difficult for you to maintain a true course through these treacherous, and sometimes impassioned waters. But that is what being a safety director is all about: using data and facts to come to a conclusion that is honest and truthful, and unimpeded by pressure from others.

Your conclusion might not make everyone your best friend, but if those involved know that you have been principled and unaffected by the pressures of the decision, then, in the long term, you will succeed, and perhaps even have an easier job the next time a controversial event occurs. Everyone will begin to recognize that you are guided by ethics and principles and do not pander or cave under pressure.

Keeping pace with best scientific practices

Keeping up to date with and using the best scientific practices available are two more essential requirements of your job. Staying in touch with scientific advancements and knowledge in your area(s) of expertise is not only good practice it is smart practice.

There are, of course, a number of ways to keep up with these trends. Taking or teaching courses/lectures is a good way of accomplishing these goals. Be a part of the leading force that develops the knowledge and then applies it to help solve a problem. Consider the environmental problem created by mercury discharge from hospitals and other industries.

Over the past 10 years, there has been a growing amount of recognition and concern among environmental groups and regulators about the use of mercury and mercury-containing products and chemicals in health care institutions across the country. At first, the level of knowledge and education about where mercury might be found in a wide array of products and chemicals was minimal, especially when it came to the minute contents of mercury found in chemicals and materials as contaminants.

Now, a decade later, mercury has been found in some cleaning products, soaps, and in a number of laboratory reagents. The information about these materials began to emerge slowly as safety professionals in a number of hospitals started to ask questions, and explore and uncover the facts about mercury use and contamination.

Today, there are lists available that not only identify the products, such as certain bleaches, where mercury can be found, but also lists of substitutes that contain little or virtually no mercury in them. Based on the knowledge that has been gained, programs are in effect in many hospitals around the country to trade in their mercury-containing materials—from thermometers to cleaning solutions—and to replace them with nonmercury-containing, or very low-mercury-containing materials and chemicals.

This program has a long way to go, and the cure for the environmental problem created by mercury discharge into water is still a long way off. However, safety professionals in hospitals all across the country are not only keeping pace with and using the best scientific knowledge, they are also helping to develop that knowledge base. Keeping up with and helping to advance the scientific knowledge base is an example of how professionals in any field, not only in the safety field, should conduct themselves.

Maintaining confidentiality

Confidentiality is an issue that almost every professional deals with during his or her career. As safety director, you will be privy to an array of information about the people who work in the hospital, and about the hospital itself. For example, as you investigate incidents, you may learn about an employee's private medical report associated with the treatment he or she received as a result of an injury that must be entered into the OSHA injury log. You may learn about working conditions that are not up to par or that may even put employees at risk and ultimately need to be corrected.

Your responsibility is to maintain confidentiality about medical data or unsafe working conditions, while at the same time addressing the latter with both employees and workers to make certain that the conditions are corrected so that they do not recreate themselves. You will also have access to employee data about exposures to hazardous materials on the job. Examples of the kinds of data that safety professionals in hospitals collect include monitoring of formaldehyde, ethylene oxide, and waste anesthetic gas. While you need to share the results of this monitoring data with the affected employee and his or her supervisor in a timely fashion, you should keep the results confidential from others who do not have a need to know. In a more general sense, learn when to share data properly and when to keep the information private until and unless it is appropriate to share.

In the final analysis, you need to behave in a manner that is beyond reproach, and that follows a standard of both excellence and ethical behavior. Do your job based on up to date science and best scientific practice. Be confident in yourself and maintain your ability to perform your job with impartiality so that you can do it well and with the proper ends in sight.

Chapter 16

Closing Thoughts

This book is a compilation of the ideas and thoughts that have resulted from my experiences as the safety director at a major teaching hospital for more than 10 years. Many books have been written about what regulations need to be followed or how to comply with Joint Commission standards. Both are very laudable goals, no doubt, but both have been replicated in many forms over the past several years. This book was written with a different goal in mind: Help give the hospital safety manager or safety director a leg up on the often long and confusing learning curve that his or her assumption of the job demands.

Today, unlike ever before, your role is a critical part of the overall support of all hospital functions. The individuals who become the safety directors of hospitals often come from a wide range of backgrounds and a wide range of experiences. In the average hospital in America, the 200- to 250-bed hospital, it is frequently a nurse, infection control nurse, or risk manager who is chosen to oversee the safety management of the facility.

The individual is selected due to his or her experience with some aspect of safety, employee injury, or insurance. Yet many of these people have a long road ahead as they take over the reins of hospital safety. Even if the candidates who are chosen have a great deal of experience in their area of expertise, it will not prepare them for what they will encounter as the safety director.

The expectations of employees, patients, visitors, and the neighbors of the hospital, as well as the regulatory agencies who oversee hospitals, have changed dramatically in the last 15 to 20 years. Hospitals are no longer regarded as comforting places run by benevolent leaders who would never do harm. The nature of health care today and an awakened realization of the potential hazards in the hospital have changed the perception that everyone has about health care facilities.

Interestingly, many of the hazards—real or imagined—in health care facilities fall under your jurisdiction. It is your job to monitor the exposures to those hazards, develop programs to help reduce those hazards, and ensure that those hazards do not escape the confines of the hospital to affect the air or water of the local neighborhood.

Your job is complex and challenging. You must be familiar with all of the regulations and know what is required to comply with them. You must also prepare employees at all levels of the health care facility to understand the requirements and comply with them. You must help the leaders and administrators develop programs that will result in a safe workplace for the employees. You must do this even while many of the procedures that are performed are potentially harmful.

If chemicals, gases, and radioactive materials are not properly handled or disposed of, such as radioactive agents during therapy or nitrous oxide during surgery, both employees and others could be put in harm's way. In addition, you often sit in the middle of controversy, pulled in different directions by the special needs and desires of the various departments.

This book looks at my thoughts and insights into the demands placed upon you. It is hoped that this book will help you avoid some of the job's pitfalls so that you can interact effectively with all the people, including staff, administrators, and regulators with whom you come into contact. The book was written to assist new or inexperienced safety directors achieve the goals of their position—a safe and healthful work environment, compliance with the regulations, and better cooperation with all members of the hospital in promoting these goals.

Good habits that you need to develop

Good habits will help you work more effectively and be more productive. You are a member of a group of professions where burnout or frustration can cut short a career. There are never any guarantees, of course, that the work will make you happy. However, many studies have shown that safety professionals are typically very satisfied with the work they do, overall.

Below are some suggestions that could help you be more productive and also help you avoid some of the burnout and frustration that could alter your career:

1. Always be honest about the problems you see and why you think there need to be changes.

2. Develop open working relationships with employees at all levels of the organization.

3. Do not become a preacher or crusader.

4. Maintain your availability to everyone—by phone, by e-mail, by personal contact.

5. Remember that sometimes goals are not achieved in one day and that not everyone will be convinced immediately of the need for a policy, program, or change in the way things are done.

6. Do not fret. You cannot win every discussion or every battle every day. Sometimes you will lose, but live to fight another day.

7. Keep up with the many things that are going on in your field. Read, read, and read!

8. Attend at least one professional seminar a year.

9. Keep abreast of the ongoing issues throughout the hospital, even if they do not appear to directly affect safety.

10. Develop resources in other departments to share the safety responsibility.

11. Do not "do" safety for people; teach them how to "do" safety, with your help, for themselves.

12. Don't put off that annual vacation